JACQU — HART

THE
COMPLETE
2-DAY
FASTING
DIET

Delicious. Easy To Make.
140 New Low-Calorie Recipes

From The Bestselling Author Of *The 5:2 Bikini Diet*

To all my dear family and friends who have joined me
on my incredible dieting adventure.

HarperThorsons
An imprint of HarperCollins*Publishers*
77–85 Fulham Palace Road
London W6 8JB

www.harpercollins.co.uk

First published by HarperThorsons 2014

3 5 7 9 10 8 6 4 2

Text © Jacqueline Whitehart 2014

Jacqueline Whitehart asserts her moral right to be
identified as the author of this work.

Photography © Claire Winfield
Food stylist: Rachel Wood
Prop stylist: Lucy Harvey

A catalogue record for this book is
available from the British Library.

PB ISBN: 978-0-00-755079-1
UK EB ISBN: 978-0-00-755379-2

Printed and bound in Great Britain by Clays Ltd, St Ives plc

CONTENTS

INTRODUCTION

The 2-Day Diet, otherwise known as the '5:2 Diet' or 'intermittent fasting', is taking the world by storm. Anyone can follow its simple premise that you only diet two days a week and eat healthily the rest of the time. These delicious and simple recipes are tailored to suit your lifestyle throughout the year. Cutting your calories for only two days a week couldn't be easier.

When I got back from holiday in August 2012 I knew it was time to lose some weight. A holiday diet of fish and chips and ice cream had left me feeling stodgy and jiggly in all the wrong places. I'd tried many diets before and never stuck to them. But as soon as I heard about the 2-Day Diet I just knew it was for me. Diet only two days a week – what's not to like? I can honestly say that I have never looked back.

With the 2-Day Diet I reached my target weight within six months and I now maintain my weight by dieting just one day a week. I have noticed other changes too. My body shape and with it my body confidence has changed. I'm not pencil thin but I'm happy and comfortable in my skin. I have got bags of energy – a definite plus when I'm chasing after my three children. Finally, the 2-Day Diet has re-invigorated my love of food and cooking. By awakening real hunger on diet days, I taste and savour every delicious mouthful of my food. On my normal days, I don't worry about food yet I eat healthily, cooking proper easy meals for myself and my family.

The recipes here are tailored to how real people eat throughout the year. In the winter, I want hot food all the time: casseroles and soups are the order of the day. Yet in summer the food I eat is totally different: I want salads and grilled meats.

Like everyone I know, I am obsessed with the weather in the UK. The sunshine (or lack of it) is forever intertwined with how I feel and what I eat.

This cookbook is about embracing the changing seasons and enjoying your food whatever the weather. The recipes are all low calorie and suitable for diet days, yet are designed to be enjoyed on any day of the week.

I hope you enjoy cooking and eating my recipes as much as I enjoyed creating them.

Find more of my recipes on my blog at www.52recipes.co.uk

Or get in touch via twitter @52DietRecipes or my Facebook page. I'm looking forward to hearing your success stories!

Yours,

Jacqueline

Jacqueline Whitehart, October 2013

GETTING STARTED

The 2-Day Diet is a diet you can stick to. People everywhere are finding that this great new diet has life-changing results. You only diet two days a week. This means that on five days a week you don't need to worry or think about food all the time. What other diet allows you puddings and nights out and still gives you amazing results? I love it and I think you will too.

How it works

On two non-consecutive days a week, follow a calorie-restricted diet. That's the jump-start. It means:

- 500 calories for women
- 600 calories for men

On the other five days, eat three healthy balanced meals a day.

A TYPICAL WEEK

MON	TUES	WED	THURS	FRI	SAT	SUN
Diet	Normal & healthy	Normal & healthy	Diet	Normal & healthy	Normal & healthy	Normal & healthy
500 (women) 600 (men)			500 (women) 600 (men)			

Why it works

By markedly trimming down your calories two days a week (you are eating one-quarter of the standard amount on those two days) you can expect 0.5–0.9kg (1–2lb) a week weight loss. When you have less food on those two days, you really recognise hunger signals. We are so used to eating whenever we feel like it. We are never quite hungry when we eat, and never quite full when we stop. These two lower calorie days help you establish those signals for life.

Your two restricted calorie days are lean protein and veggie based, for adequate nutrition, and so you don't have to worry about getting enough protein for your body's needs.

The most amazing difference between the 2-Day Diet and other diets is that when you drastically reduce your calories on the two diet days you are burning off body fat instead of muscle.

The strict two days help you learn to recognise biological hunger and fullness. As you are eating less food you will be actively hungry for your next meal. You will learn to savour every mouthful.

You will appreciate the extra guilt-free calories on your healthy days. Appreciating and enjoying your food gives you a huge boost and is the heart of the 2-Day Diet.

Change in lifestyle

The 2-Day Diet is not a quick fix. The aim is to establish good long-term eating habits. The two diet days are a jump-start for weight loss, but it is not a miracle diet. The diet days boost your weight loss by 0.9–1.4kg (2–3lb) a week at the start of the diet, reducing to about 0.5kg (1lb) a week subsequently. The real change comes through eating healthily on your other five days. Eating three healthy meals a day and cutting out the junk food will enable you to maintain the weight loss from the diet days. You should feel better in yourself and full of energy.

The simplicity of the 2-Day Diet is extremely compelling and it is so easy to get started. As you progress with the diet, you will find that the key to long-term success is how you manage your diet days. If you don't eat the right food, then you feel starving and unable to cope: this makes you far more likely to cheat or give up. I remember on my first day, I had a large glass of orange juice at breakfast time. This 'wasted' 100 or so calories which I was in desperate need of by dinner time. By eating the right food and not eating 'empty calories' you can eat enough to keep going throughout the day. This is the core of this cookbook. You can find the right food to eat for every day and it is always tasty and filling. If your diet day is pain-free then you can stick with the diet, change your lifestyle and ultimately your figure.

THE JUMP-START –
YOUR LOW-CALORIE DAYS

A little bit of planning will help your first few diet days fly by. Follow these steps to ease you through your first two days:

1. Decide which days you are going to diet during the week.
Remember the days must be non-consecutive. Think about what you've got on in your schedule. The best days are busy but not social ones. So pick your boring days and you will be fine.

2. How many meals are you going to eat on your diet days?
Three small meals **OR** breakfast and dinner **OR** lunch and dinner.

3. Use the appropriate meal planner as a guide.
Set out what you are going to eat. Buy and prepare your food in advance.

What kind of dieter are you?

Use this handy guide to help you work out the best days to diet and the best times to eat during the day.

If you work 9–5

- Try to diet on the same days each week – try Monday and Thursday.
- Eat a filling breakfast and make it through to an early dinner as soon as you come home from work.
- Work through your lunchtime or go for a brisk, refreshing walk.
- Plan and prepare your evening meal in advance so that it is quick and easy to cook when you get home.

If you are single

- Plan your diet days for days when you are busy but have no social engagements, especially if they involve food or drink.
- The days you diet can be flexible so you can choose different days each week – check your calendar and plan accordingly.
- Prepare your food in advance. Cook batches and freeze in individual portions. Then you will have a perfect meal ready in minutes when you get home from work.
- Eat one or two small meals or snacks during the day, having most of your calories in the evening.
- Keep busy on diet day evenings – try out a hobby or go for a walk.

If you are a full-time mum

- Choose your diet days so they are your busiest days when you and the kids are out and about.
- Eat three small meals at the same time as your children.
- Prepare your food in advance so it is ready at the same time as their food.
- Eat your main meal as an early tea with your family. You may find you can eat the same meal – just without the carbs.

If you are dieting as a couple

- Try to make sure you both diet on the same days. Consult your diaries and stick to the same plan.
- Men can eat an extra 100 calories per day, so they can have a little extra for breakfast or lunch.
- Plan to sit down and eat your evening meal together.
- Go to the cinema or for a walk together on the evenings of your diet days.

If you are a serial diet failure

- Plan out your diet days carefully. Come up with a schedule and stick to it.
- Try dieting on a Monday and Wednesday as that way you will get your diet days out of the way as quickly as possible.
- If you are struggling with motivation on a diet day, remember why the 2-Day Diet is different – tomorrow you can eat normally with no guilt.
- Everyone finds some days harder than others. But as you get used to the diet it gets easier and easier.
- If you fall off the wagon one week you can always try again next week – don't give up!

What to expect on your first diet day

If you are feeling a little nervous about your first day: don't be. Think positive and it will fly by.

Your first day may be the hardest. This is because you may never have allowed yourself to be properly hungry before and your body is telling you that this is wrong. Rest assured, it is natural to feel hungry. Ease your hunger pangs with a calorie-free drink or go for a walk.

The most important thing to remember is that it is only one day and tomorrow you can eat like a king. Feel proud of yourself.

If you are hungry you are actively losing weight. Revel in a real sense of achievement.

Headaches and light-headedness

If you are reading this on your first diet day then I suspect you are feeling one or other of these common symptoms for the first day. Not everyone gets these but if you are one of them, then read on for some simple ways to combat them and get through the day.

Headaches are a common problem in the first few days of the 2-Day Diet. I believe the main cause of this is a change in caffeine intake. If you normally have a few cups of tea and coffee then a headache is almost a given if you cut down. But as this diet is not about caffeine-reduction and you are most likely to go back to your normal intake tomorrow, then any headache you have today is in vain.

Think about what your average caffeine intake is on a regular day and try and have a similar amount of drinks on a diet day too. I normally incorporate my normal skinny latte and two cups of tea into every diet day. But you do need to count the calories so if your normal caffeinated drinks are too calorific for a diet day then you need to swap to something else. Any coffee drink without milk has negligible calories, think Americano or Espresso. If you prefer a milky drink then make sure you use skimmed milk and don't overdo the milk. Also worth trying are drinks such as green tea, which is mildly caffeinated and, of course, diet colas are an option.

Drink	approx caffeine content
Espresso, Latte, Americano, Cappuccino (small or medium sizes containing one shot of espresso)	75mg
Filter coffee or flat white coffee	110mg
Instant coffee	90mg
Tea (will vary with brewing time)	50mg
Green tea	40mg
Diet coke	42mg
Coke/Coke zero	32mg
Pepsi Max	69mg
Diet Pepsi	35mg
40g (1½oz) bar dark chocolate	6mg

As a general guide, your caffeine intake should be below 500mg per day. But if you are sensitive to caffeine or suffer from headaches, restlessness or anxiety you should consider dropping this to less than 250mg. If you have trouble sleeping, try not to consume any caffeine after 3pm. This is because caffeine has a half-life of eight hours. If it is consumed after 3pm, it may still be affecting you at 11pm. For the purposes of the diet, you should be trying to maintain your standard consumption of caffeine so as to maintain a feeling of well-being over your diet day.

Light-headedness or dizziness can be a problem, particularly on your first diet day. This is your body 'rebelling' against the diet and saying it can't cope when really it can! In fact, studies have shown that tests done on people suffering from a 'blood sugar crash' have actually had normal blood sugar levels. The first thing to do if you get a wave of light-headedness is to move about and get some fresh air if possible. The wave might well pass in 15 minutes.

If this is still your first week of the diet and you are finding that one or other of these symptoms is limiting your ability to function normally, then you should eat something small and filling. Ideally go for about 100 calories, perhaps a small banana or a Ryvita with a light spread of soft cheese. On these days you will eat 100 calories more in total – so that is 600 for women and 700 for men.

Don't let it put you off, and you will find the next day easier. Your body adapts quickly and after two weeks it should no longer impact on your feelings of well-being.

Finally, if you are a new starter, the great news is your weight loss in the first week or two is at its most dramatic. After two to three weeks it will stabilise. So push on through, you will see the results on the scales almost immediately.

Ten top tips to stay strong on your diet days

1 Know exactly what you are going to eat and stick to it.
2 Keep busy all the time.
3 Stay out of the kitchen and away from the smell of food.
4 Choose a guilt-free drink or nibble when you feel the urge to eat.
5 Tell yourself you can always eat [fill in the blank] tomorrow.
6 If you feel a wave of hunger, get some fresh air and it will soon pass.
7 Clear out your cupboards and fridge of tempting treats.
8 Take it one day at a time – each day gets easier.
8 Savour every mouthful of the food you eat.
10 Get on the scales the morning after your first fast day – you will have lost weight... but how much?

Guilt-free snacking: 10 foods less than 10 calories

Please note calories are approximate here.
1 Five slices of yellow pepper
2 Diet cola or lemonade
3 Two sticks of celery
4 Fruit tea
5 Five radishes
6 Small cup of hot Bovril made with 1 level tsp Bovril
7 Three cherry tomatoes
8 Sparkling water with ice and lemon
9 Two strawberries
10 Low-cal jelly

DIET DAY PLANNER

You can download and print this planner from
www.52recipes.co.uk

PLANNER FOR:

WEIGHT BEFORE
(step on the scales the evening before your diet day)

MEAL	FOOD EATEN	CALORIES
BREAKFAST		
LUNCH		
DINNER		
OTHER		
TOTAL		

**Day completed
without problems?**   YES / NO

How difficult was it?
(Score out of 10)

WEIGHT AFTER
(step on the scales the evening before your diet day)

TOTAL WEIGHT LOSS

EVERYDAY EATING FOR YOUR FIVE HEALTHY DAYS

The absolutely amazing thing about the 2-Day Diet is that you only have to be on a diet for two days. Yet to get the best results you need to make healthy choices every day of the week. There is plenty of good news for your healthy days:

- Treats are allowed.
- You should not count calories.
- Do not feel guilty if you eat something naughty.

Change your attitude to food and you will make positive lifestyle changes.

- Be aware of what you eat
- Choose three healthy balanced meals
- Eat less snacks
- Limit your food intake

By following these simple guidelines you will notice improvements in your well-being as well as your waistline.

Look for your weak spots. Is it the office treats table? Boozy drinks after work? Junk food snacking? Evening cravings? Find what you think is your worst offence and make a conscious effort to curb this every day of the week. I think one of the best ways is to set yourself a specific goal and reward.

Eat well

Eating well on your five healthy days doesn't need to be hard. Try and cook real food every day of the week. Choose simple recipes that are balanced and low in fat. Try not to snack too much. Most importantly, banish the junk food as much as you can.

Top tips!

- Remember to eat three meals a day with not too many snacks.
- Cook food such as soups and stews and freeze in one or two person portions.
- Make a 7-day plan (see page 16) to incorporate your diet days and healthy days.
- Use the simple recipes in this book for healthy days too. Just add some extra carbohydrates such as rice and potatoes.
- Prepare food in advance if you can.
- Take a salad or last night's leftovers in a lunchbox, rather than buying sandwiches for lunch.

Ten ways to be good AND have fun

1 Have set alcohol-free days every week.
2 Remove all biscuits from the house but vow to make your own at the weekend.
3 Go crisp-free.
4 Allow yourself a 'treat' on a Friday if you have been good all week.
5 Give yourself a time and/or drinks limit when you go out.
6 Read the ingredients and calories of any junk food before you eat it.
7 Switch from beer to spirits with a diet mixer.
8 Walk or cycle instead of taking the car.
9 Go to the greengrocer instead of the supermarket and be inspired to make something simple and different.
10 Make a home-made takeaway, such as Chicken tikka masala (see page 214) or Chinese chicken stir-fry (see page 165).

Sample 7-day meal planner: Spring

Here is a sample weekly planner, showing both diet days and normal days. Diet days are Monday and Thursday. The season is Spring.

	Breakfast	Lunch	Dinner	Other	Cals
Mon Diet day	1 slice Fruity bran loaf (page 39) 156 *cals*	Spicy sweet potato soup (page 42) 125 *cals*	Cajun fried chicken (page 52) and small salad 253 *cals*	1 med (100g/3½oz) banana (MEN only) 95 *cals*	**498** **(593 men)**
Tues Normal day	Scrambled eggs on toast	Spicy sweet potato soup (page 42) with a hunk of baguette	Spring chicken stew (page 71) with mashed potato (freeze half)	1 slice Fruity bran loaf (page 39), yogurt, fresh fruit	
Wed Normal day	2 slices Fruity bran loaf (page 39) with butter and jam	Smoked fish chowder (page 56) with bread (freeze 3 portions)	Grilled lamb in fresh parsley and mint sauce (page 63) with new potatoes and green veg	Fresh fruit, few squares dark chocolate	
Thurs Diet day	1 Ryvita (35) with 1 Babybel Light (53), sliced 98 *cals*	Garlicky King prawns (page 47) 134 *cals*	Grilled lamb in fresh parsley and mint sauce (241) (page 63) and 50g (1¾oz) baby spinach (12) 253 *cals*	40g (scant ¼ cup) couscous with lamb (MEN only) 91 *cals*	**485** **(576 men)**

	Breakfast	Lunch	Dinner	Other	Cals
Fri Normal day	Power up breakfast (page 54)	Garlic prawn wrap with salad	Vietnamese yellow curry (page 64) with basmati rice	Sweet 'treat'	
Sat Normal day	Sausage, egg and mushrooms on toast	Cheat's Caesar salad (page 44)	Spring chicken stew (page 71) with baked potato	2 glasses wine	
Sun Normal day	Sausage sandwich	Smoked fish chowder (page 56) with bread	Vietnamese yellow curry (page 64) with rice and naan bread	Yogurt, few squares dark chocolate	

All of the recipes can be found in the Spring chapter of this cookbook (see pages 29–77). Take a look at the Plate fillers section (see page 223) for more ideas of good carbohydrates to include in your normal days. Notice how I have made sure no food is wasted. I have made two person recipes and eaten the second portion for lunch or dinner, either the next day or on subsequent days. I have also made a batch of soup and frozen portions for later in the week.

Shopping list for full seven days

Meat and fish

2 × 90g (3¼oz) lean lamb leg
  steaks

50g (1¾oz) streaky bacon

2 skinless, boneless chicken
  thighs

400g (14oz) skinless chicken
  breasts

400g (14oz) skinless smoked
  haddock

200g (7oz) raw king prawns
  (shrimp)

4 sausages

Fruit and veg

2 small sweet potatoes

2 large potatoes

700g (1½lb) new potatoes

2 Little Gem (Boston) lettuce

1 cos (Romaine) lettuce

Bag baby spinach

Bag mixed salad leaves

Cucumber

2 medium tomatoes

Cherry tomatoes

6 spring onions (scallions)

5 leeks

Mushrooms

1 celery stick

1 lemongrass stalk

1 green chilli

Frozen peas

Garlic

3 lemons

1 banana (men only)

Dairy

900ml (4 cups) skimmed milk

4 eggs

Babybel Lights

10g (2 tsp) butter

10g (2 tsp) Parmesan cheese

Low-fat plain yogurt

Fruit yogurt pots

Storecupboard

Wholemeal (wholewheat)
  bread

1 baguette

Ryvitas

Wraps

All-Bran

Caster (superfine) sugar

Sultanas (golden raisins)

Dried apricots

Dried figs

Dates

Wholemeal self-raising
  (wholewheat self-rising)
  flour

Couscous (men only)

Basmati rice

Naan bread

Porridge (rolled) oats

Granola

Olive oil

Sunflower oil

Extra virgin olive oil

Black peppercorns

Cornflour (cornstarch)

Vegetable stock (bouillon) cubes

Fish stock

Tomato ketchup

Extra-light mayonnaise

White wine vinegar

Dijon mustard

Dry (hard) cider

1 can light coconut milk

1 can anchovies

Jar capers

Black olives

Dark chocolate

Medium curry powder, smoked paprika, ground cumin, cumin seeds, hot paprika, cayenne pepper, ground turmeric, ground ginger

Dried thyme, dried oregano, dried mixed herbs, bay leaf

Fresh mint, fresh tarragon, flat-leaf parsley, fresh coriander (cilantro)

Salt and pepper

Light oil spray

THE FASTING PHENOMENON

The 2-Day Diet is fast becoming one of the most popular diets worldwide. In the UK it is the most talked about diet of 2013 and has spread all around the world. It is incredibly popular in Ireland, Sweden and South Africa, to name just a few.

But why is it proving so successful? I think there are two unique draws of the diet which make people choose it AND stick to it.

Firstly it is the diet's **simplicity** that is its main selling point. You can easily describe how to do the diet in one sentence and anyone can go and get started straight away. You don't need to buy special foods or pay anyone any money.

The second point is the 2-Day Diet's **long-term success rate**. People who start the diet are more likely to stick to it than other diets. This is because you are not dieting every day, meaning you can still enjoy life's pleasures five days a week.

Another reason why so many people love the diet is that it really can burn those last few pounds like no other diet. When you diet normally, the body will always use the simplest energy stores first. This means that you will always burn off the food you have just eaten rather than the fat on your hips. When you do the 2-Day Diet, on your diet days you enter a semi-fasting state and your blood glucose levels fall. This triggers the release of metabolic fuels from the body's stores of fat. The 2-Day Diet is therefore one of the most effective diets for burning fat.[1]

Health benefits

The majority of people following the 2-Day Diet are interested primarily in weight loss. Losing weight and reducing your BMI obviously has plenty of health benefits. But on top of the health benefits of losing weight there are also indicators that this type of weight loss has advantages over and above other forms of diet.

Areas where intermittent fasting seems to bring additional benefits are diabetes, heart disease and Alzheimer's prevention. Research into intermittent fasting is ongoing and 2013 has brought some interesting new topics to light.

The most research has been done into diabetes and heart health. Does intermittent fasting reduce the risk of diabetes and cardiovascular markers for heart disease? A review of current research [2] suggests that limiting calories in this way can reverse type 2 diabetes and has the potential to be cardio-protective.

On first glance the link between being overweight and Alzheimer's does not seem obvious. But when you note that more and more scientists now see Alzheimer's as just another form of diabetes, then things begin to fall in to place. This has grave implications worldwide. The prospect of an Alzheimer's epidemic on the scale of the current worldwide obesity epidemic is extremely alarming. Yet there is growing evidence to suggest that Alzheimer's disease is type 3 diabetes [3]. If this proves to be true, then there is reason to believe that intermittent fasting and the weight loss associated with it will offer some protection against Alzheimer's in later years.

There is countless anecdotal evidence to suggest that combining intermittent fasting and exercise maximises weight loss and body changes. A new study [4] published in *Obesity* in July 2013 certainly strengthens this belief. In the study of 64 obese individuals, those combining intermittent fasting and exercise lost the most weight. Over 12 weeks, the average weight loss of those doing both was 6kg (13lb); of those just doing intermittent fasting the weight loss was 3kg (6.6lb) and of those just doing exercise, it was 1kg (2.2lb).

TODAY, TOMORROW, FOREVER?

The 2-Day Diet is not a miracle fad diet, promising extreme weight loss in a short period of time. More and more people are realising that intermittent fasting is a lifestyle choice. It works and can comfortably be maintained for as long as it's needed. In fact, many people, myself included, choose to continue with one diet day a week even after optimum weight loss has been achieved.

You should expect to lose 0.9–2kg (2–4lb) a week in the first two weeks, dropping to 0.5–0.9kg (1–2lb) a week as your body gets used to the diet. Exactly how much you lose depends on your starting weight and your choices on your five normal days.

If you feel that your weight loss has plateaued and you haven't lost any weight for at least two weeks then you may have hit the wall in terms of weight loss. But don't worry, there are ways to kick-start your weight loss again.

1. The simplest and most common cause of a weight-loss plateau is an increase of calories on your five healthy days. Are there a few too many treats creeping in? Keep a food diary. Just tracking your food honestly should help you to cut back. Look at the snacks and junk food and see which ones should be cut out.

2. Increase your diet days to three days a week. Your body may have adapted to two diet days so by having three diet days a week, you are mixing things up and giving yourself optimum weight-loss conditions.

3. Take a week off. I know this is counterintuitive, but allowing your metabolism to rest (while eating healthily to ensure you don't gain weight) should improve your chances of success when you re-start the diet.

Most importantly, don't give up! If you have hit a wall and are having doubts that the diet is working for you, please stop worrying. As you near your target weight, you will find that the amount of weight you lose each week will decrease. And the small drop in weight may not be accurately recorded on the scales. If you are still following the diet and eating healthily then you will shift those last few pounds. You may find that you are changing shape even if this is not reflected on the scales. Keep off the scales and only jump on every two to three weeks.

Low-carb 2-Day Diet

If you get bored of counting calories or find it difficult on your diet days, you may want to try this new variation suggested by Michelle Harvie and others from the Genesis breast cancer prevention centre.

On your two diet days, follow a very low-carb diet (think 'Atkins') but do not count calories. Their incipient research [5] suggests that this is at least as effective for weight loss and other health markers as the restricted calorie approach.

WHAT TO DO IF...

These are all genuine questions that people have asked via Facebook www.facebook.com/52DietRecipes or Twitter @52DietRecipes. If you have got a question that's not listed here, I'd love to help if I can.

If your plans change and you suddenly find yourself in the pub on a diet day

Don't panic! You have got two choices. Do you break the diet or not? Having a drink and breaking the diet would mean that the effort you have put in during the day would be lost and you'd have to schedule another diet day later in the week. If it's the evening and you have already got through most of the day, is it really worth giving up on the diet day? You could have a water, a diet coke or diet tonic water without adding any extra calories.

If you're starving and there's nothing in the cupboards

Eggs, baked beans and soups are your friends here. All are filling and you should find the calorie content on the box. If you don't have any of these in your house, all will be available from your nearest supermarket or convenience store.

If you need/want to exercise on your diet day

Sometimes you will find that you have to do exercise on your diet day. The problem with exercising is that it burns calories and makes you hungry, meaning that you are more likely to struggle with your diet day. Sadly you cannot add on the calories that you burn during exercise to your calorie intake for the day. If you do need to exercise on a diet day, try to do it before you eat in the morning. Light exercise in the evening can also be a distraction from hunger. Try to avoid exercising in the afternoon as this will make you very hungry and most likely to falter.

What is the best type of exercise to do on my healthy days?

I would recommend any aerobic exercise that increases your breathing and heart rate as being best for weight loss. Walking, jogging, cycling, swimming or tennis are all good to get your heart rate up. Try to exercise three times a week for at least 45 minutes each time.

If you find a diet day is proving next to impossible

Sometimes this happens to the best of us. For all sorts of reasons – stress, hormonal, lack of sleep – we can find a diet day particularly hard. You **are** allowed to give up on a day if it is truly dreadful.

It is always worth assessing what is causing it to be so hard and trying to see if it is worth pushing on through. Late afternoon is often a time when we feel at our weakest. If you can bring your evening meal forward or have a small snack at that time, you may find you get over the hump. Remember that the sacrifices you have made already during the day will be wasted if you stop.

Try counting the number of hours until bedtime and make sure you get an early night.

If you give up entirely on a diet day, don't beat yourself up about it. Allow yourself tomorrow off and re-attempt the following day. If you still manage to fit two diet days into your week, then the week has been a success.

If you are on holiday

I think it is very hard to follow the 2-Day Diet when you are on holiday. If you have been dieting for weeks beforehand, then I would say that it is time to relax and enjoy your hard work. To avoid putting on too much weight, try to still be sensible when you can. Eat a big breakfast (especially if it's free!), eat healthy snacks or a light lunch and enjoy your dinner.

If you're cooking for other (unsympathetic!) people

If you have got a partner or family who are not dieting then you need to make sure you can accommodate everyone's needs without much fuss. The easiest way to deal with this common problem is to cook the same meal for everyone. Just serve everyone else's meal with plenty of extra carbohydrates. If it's not possible to all eat the same thing, then at the very least try to eat at the same time. There's nothing worse than watching other people eat when you're starving.

If you feel that your weight loss has plateaued

It is natural for your weight loss to level out after a few weeks on the 2-Day Diet. The high weight loss that you experience when you start the diet can only be maintained for two to three weeks.

After that, at the same time as it gets easier and you get into a rhythm, the weight loss will diminish. This is normal and healthy. The extreme early weight loss cannot be maintained. If you have a lot of weight to lose, then you will hopefully find that the weight loss flattens out at about 0.9kg (2lb) a week. If you are nearer your target weight, your expected loss will be about 0.5kg (1lb) a week.

If you are not losing any weight while still following the diet plan, then you should look at what you are eating on the five normal days. You may be eating too much. Indeed this is the most likely cause of a plateau. Make a food diary for your healthy days and be a bit stricter with yourself. Most importantly steer away from the biscuit tin and any junk food.

SPRING

SPRING RECIPES

Under 200 calories

Nutty banana energy bars

Fruity bran loaf

Roasted parsnip soup

Creamy pea and mint soup

Spicy sweet potato soup

Super easy coleslaw

Cheat's Caesar salad

Celeriac remoulade with smoked trout

Japanese-style sake prawn salad

Garlicky king prawns

Saffron 'rice' cauliflower

Oven-baked vegetable fritters

Courgette ribbons with tomato and chorizo sauce

Quick tomato and mangetout curry

Cajun fried chicken

Garlic grilled chicken

Under 300 calories

Power up breakfast
Baked eggs with ham and tomato
Smoked fish chowder
Quick tomato haddock
Purple sprouting broccoli with creamy caper sauce
Patatas bravas
Warming leek 'pasta' with olives
Asian-style stir-fried beef and mushrooms
Grilled lamb in fresh parsley and mint sauce
Vietnamese yellow curry
Slow-baked chicken rolls in tomato sauce
Blueberry fool
Baked banana with dark chocolate
Crème de menthe pudding with chocolate crunch

Under 400 calories

Paprika chicken salad
Spring chicken stew
Grilled lamb with tangy lemon couscous
Spicy lamb keema
Slow-cooked stuffed cabbage rolls
Creamy purple sprouting broccoli with Parma ham

BE INSPIRED BY THE SEASON OF HOPE

Spring is all about hope. After a long winter of cold grey days, all you want is some sun and a few green shoots. You probably want to ring the changes when it comes to food too. Are you bored of stews and soups and crave something lighter and greener?

You may find that you and your body are eager for transformation, but what about the weather? In March it may feel like the depths of winter, with snow still on the ground, but try to ignore the weather and listen to your body. Eat healthily, even on days when you are not dieting. Do some exercise: a gentle swim on any day of the week will re-invigorate you. Most importantly, if the sun does pop its head out, get outside and feel the sun on your face.

Spring recipes embrace the change but also the vagaries of the season. There are not many seasonal vegetables available and it is traditionally 'the hungry gap'. Try out some unusual salads, explore what's in your storecupboard, and experiment with the vegetables that are in season. Purple sprouting broccoli is an amazingly tasty green vegetable. Available from late February, it has a lot more to offer than its more familiar cousin. Spring is also the time to enjoy some tender lamb – a lean lamb steak can easily be incorporated into a diet day.

Let's not get carried away and keep some soups and stews in reserve for the bleakest days. If you can keep a few portions of warming soups stocked in your freezer then you are fully prepared to face the challenges that spring can bring.

Stock the freezer, count the daffodils and celebrate when the clocks change. It is a season of preparation. If you stick to the diet through the spring you'll be ready and waiting for the beach.

Menu plans for diet days

Use these planners to inspire your cooking on diet days. It's amazing how much good food you can eat for under 500–600 calories.

Just work out whether you want three small meals/breakfast and dinner/lunch and dinner on your diet days and choose the right planner for you. If you need more help working out which plan is right for you have a look at *What kind of dieter are you?* (see page 6).

Feel free to swap a recipe for another with a similar calorie content if necessary.

MENU PLANS FOR DIET DAYS: WOMEN (SPRING)

WOMEN: 3 SMALL MEALS

	Breakfast	Lunch	Dinner	Cals
Day 1	Nutty banana energy bar (page 37) 118 cals	Spicy sweet potato soup (page 42) 125 cals	Warming leek 'pasta' with olives (page 61) (233) 1 small satsuma (18) 251 cals	494
Day 2	Nutty banana energy bar (page 37) 118 cals	Cheat's Caesar salad (page 44) 143 cals	Quick tomato haddock (page 57) (225) 50g (1¾oz) spinach (12) 237 cals	498

WOMEN: BREAKFAST AND DINNER

	Breakfast	Dinner	Cals
Day 1	Power up breakfast (page 54) 219 cals	Asian-style stir-fried beef and mushrooms (page 62) 267 cals	486
Day 2	Baked eggs with ham and tomato (page 55) 251 cals	Patatas bravas (page 59) 248 cals	499

WOMEN: LUNCH AND DINNER

	Lunch	Dinner	Cals
Day 1	Garlicky King prawns (page 47) 134 cals	Spring chicken stew (page 71) 365 cals	499
Day 2	Creamy pea and mint soup (page 41) 151 cals	Grilled lamb with tangy lemon couscous (page 72) 314 cals	465

MENU PLANS FOR DIET DAYS: MEN (SPRING)

MEN: 3 SMALL MEALS

	Breakfast	Lunch	Dinner	Cals
Day 1	Nutty banana energy bar (page 37) 118 cals	Oven-baked vegetable fritters (page 49) 149 cals	Creamy purple sprouting broccoli with Parma ham (page 77) 337 cals	604
Day 2	Nutty banana energy bar (page 37) 118 cals	Warming leek 'pasta' with olives (page 61) 233 cals	Grilled lamb in fresh parsley and mint sauce (page 63) 241 cals	592

MEN: BREAKFAST AND DINNER

	Breakfast	Dinner	Cals
Day 1	Baked eggs with ham and tomato (page 55) 251 cals	Cajun fried chicken (page 52) (193) 200g (7oz) new potatoes (4 small) (140) 335 cals	586
Day 2	Power up breakfast (page 54) 219 cals	Vietnamese yellow curry (page 64) (251) 40g (scant ¼ cup) basmati rice (144) 395 cals	614

MEN: LUNCH AND DINNER

	Lunch	Dinner	Cals
Day 1	Roasted parsnip soup (page 40) (139) Slice of wholemeal (wholewheat) bread (110) 249 cals	Paprika chicken salad (page 70) (300) 100g (scant ¾ cup) strawberries (27) 327 cals	576
Day 2	Japanese-style sake prawn salad (page 46) 140 cals	Spicy lamb keema (page 74) (316) 40g (scant ¼ cup) brown rice (143) 459 cals	599

SPRING RECIPES

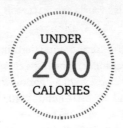

UNDER
200
CALORIES

Nutty banana energy bars

118 calories each

Using quinoa as well as oats in these bars reduces the calorie count and adds a slight nutty taste.

Makes 16 bars   Preparation time: 20 minutes   Cook time: 50 minutes
Vegetarian

light oil spray (3 cals)
....
50g (¼ cup) quinoa, well rinsed (154 cals)
....
170g (2 cups) porridge (rolled) oats (605 cals)
....
1 tsp ground cinnamon
....
1 tsp baking powder (7 cals)
....
1 tbsp desiccated (dry unsweetened) coconut (49 cals)
....
pinch of salt
....
50g (¹/₃ cup) dried cranberries (162 cals)
....
30g (¼ cup) pecans, chopped (207 cals)
....
3 medium very ripe bananas, mashed (356 cals)
....
1 large egg, beaten (91 cals)
....

continued

50g (4 tbsp) maple syrup (131 cals)

1 tbsp sunflower oil (99 cals)

2 tsp vanilla extract (24 cals)

- Line a 25 × 25cm (10 × 10in) baking tray (cookie sheet) with two pieces of baking parchment, forming a cross shape so that all the sides are covered and spray with light oil spray.
- Place the quinoa and 125ml (½ cup) water in a small saucepan and bring to the boil. Reduce the heat and simmer gently for 12–15 minutes or until the liquid is just absorbed. Remove from the heat and rest, covered, for 5 minutes. Transfer to a bowl and fluff with a fork. Leave to cool completely.
- Preheat the oven to 160°C/140°C fan/325°F/Gas mark 3.
- Place the oats, cinnamon, baking powder, desiccated (dry unsweetened) coconut and salt in a large bowl and mix thoroughly. Then mix in the dried cranberries and chopped pecans.
- Add the mashed bananas, beaten egg, maple syrup, oil and vanilla to the quinoa and stir until just combined. Add the banana mixture to the oat mixture and loosely mix.
- Press the batter into the prepared baking tray and bake in the oven for 35–40 minutes. Leave to cool completely in the tray.
- When cool, lift out using the baking parchment and transfer to a chopping board. Cut into 16 bars. Wrap individually in clingfilm (plastic wrap) and store in the refrigerator for up to a week. Alternatively, store in an airtight container in the freezer for up to three months.

Fruity bran loaf

156 calories (per slice)

This tasty fruit loaf is full of goodness and a favourite with kids and adults alike. It will keep for up to a week in an airtight tin and freezes well.

Makes 10 slices   Preparation time: 5 minutes, plus standing

Cook time: 35–40 minutes

Very easy, freezer-friendly

100g (1½ cups) All-Bran (or similar, but not bran flakes) (270 cals)

90g (½ cup) caster (superfine) sugar (355 cals)

100g (½ cup) sultanas (golden raisins) (275 cals)

50g (¼ cup) dried apricots, chopped (94 cals)

50g (1¾oz) dried figs, chopped (114 cals)

50g (1¾oz) dates, chopped (62 cals)

250ml (generous 1 cup) skimmed (skim) milk (80 cals)

light oil spray (3 cals)

100g (¾ cup) wholemeal self-raising (wholewheat self-rising) flour (310 cals)

- Put the All-Bran, sugar and dried fruit into a bowl and mix together well. Stir in the milk and leave to stand for 30 minutes.
- Preheat the oven to 180°C/160°C fan/350°F/Gas mark 4 and oil a loaf tin (pan) well with oil spray.
- Sift in the flour, mixing well. Pour the mixture into the prepared loaf tin (loaf pan) and bake for 35–40 minutes. Turn out of the tin immediately and leave to cool on a wire rack.

Roasted parsnip soup

139 calories

This soup is comforting with a little added zing.

Serves 4   Preparation time: 20 minutes   Cook time: 35 minutes

Vegetarian, freezer-friendly

1 tbsp olive oil (99 cals)
6 medium parsnips (about 80g/3oz each), peeled and cut into large cubes (307 cals)
salt and freshly ground black pepper
1 tsp olive oil (27 cals)
1 small onion, peeled and finely chopped (22 cals)
zest of 1 lemon (2 cals)
¼ tsp vanilla extract
500ml (generous 2 cups) vegetable stock, fresh or from 1 cube (35 cals)
200ml (generous ¾ cup) skimmed (skim) milk (64 cals)

- Preheat the oven to 190°C/170°C fan/375°F/Gas mark 5.
- Pour the 1 tablespoon olive oil over the parsnips and season generously with salt and pepper. Use your hands to toss the parsnips in the oil, making sure they are well covered.
- Spread the parsnips out over a baking tray and roast in the oven for 20 minutes.
- While the parsnips are in the oven, heat the 1 teaspoon oil in a large saucepan, add the onion and fry gently for 10 minutes until softened.
- Add the lemon zest, vanilla, stock and 100ml (scant ½ cup) water, then bring to the boil.
- Add the roasted parsnips and return to the boil. Reduce the heat, put the lid on and simmer gently for a further 15 minutes.
- Transfer to a blender and blend until smooth. Return to the pan, add the milk and stir. Reheat gently and serve.

Creamy pea and mint soup

151 calories

Serves 4   Preparation time: 5 minutes   Cook time: 20 minutes

Vegetarian, freezer-friendly

1 tbsp olive oil (99 cals)
8 spring onions (scallions), trimmed and roughly chopped (40 cals)
1 iceberg lettuce (400g/14oz), outer leaves removed and roughly chopped (52 cals)
400g (3½ cups) frozen peas (264 cals)
900ml (3½ cups) vegetable or chicken stock (fresh is best here) (70 cals)
8 fresh mint leaves
100g (scant ½ cup) low-fat Greek yogurt (80 cals)
freshly ground black pepper

- In a large saucepan, heat the oil over a low heat. Stir in the spring onions and lettuce for 1–2 minutes until the lettuce starts to wilt.
- Add the peas, stock and mint leaves. Bring to a gentle simmer and cook for 15 minutes or until all the vegetables are tender.
- Blend the soup until smooth. For an even smoother texture, pass the soup through a sieve after blending.
- Stir in the yogurt and bring back up to temperature before serving. Season with black pepper and serve.

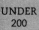

Spicy sweet potato soup

125 calories

This is a very quick and easy soup.

Serves 2   Preparation time: 5 minutes   Cook time: 20–25 minutes

Vegetarian, freezer-friendly

1 tsp olive oil (27 cals)
2 small sweet potatoes, peeled and roughly chopped (174 cals)
2 garlic cloves, peeled and crushed (6 cals)
1 tsp medium curry powder (7 cals)
½ tsp smoked paprika (3 cals)
1 tsp cornflour (cornstarch) (5 cals)
½ vegetable stock (bouillon) cube (17 cals)
1 tsp tomato ketchup (8 cals)
juice of 1 lemon (3 cals)

- Heat the oil in a saucepan, add the sweet potatoes and garlic and fry for 4–5 minutes. Sprinkle in the curry powder, paprika and cornflour (cornstarch) and stir-fry for 1 more minute.
- Add 2 tablespoons water and stir to form a paste (this is to stop the cornflour going lumpy) before adding 470ml (2 cups) water. Crumble in the stock (bouillon) cube and add the ketchup and lemon juice. Bring to the boil, then reduce the heat and simmer for 15–20 minutes or until the sweet potato is tender.
- Transfer to a blender and blend until smooth, then serve.

Super easy coleslaw

112 cals

Can be eaten on its own for a light lunch or as a low-calorie accompaniment to a meat or chicken dish.

Serves 1   Preparation time: 5 minutes

Vegetarian

1 tbsp low-fat yogurt (22 cals)
1 tbsp skimmed (skim) milk (5 cals)
pinch of salt
¼ white cabbage (200g/7oz), finely shredded (54 cals)
1 small apple, cored and thinly sliced (31 cals)

- Mix together the yogurt, milk and salt and set aside.
- Combine the cabbage and apple, then pour the dressing over and mix lightly.

Cheat's Caesar salad

143 calories

Serves 1   Preparation time: 10 minutes

Quick & easy

1 (100g/3½oz) cos (Romaine) lettuce, washed and outer leaves removed (16 cals)
2 tbsp extra-light mayonnaise (24 cals)
1 tbsp low-fat yogurt (14 cals)
1 tsp white wine vinegar (1 cals)
4 anchovy fillets, drained and chopped (24 cals)
1 tsp capers (1 cal)
10g (2 tbsp) Parmesan cheese, finely grated (42 cals)
4 large black olives (21 cals)
freshly ground black pepper

- Chop the lettuce into ribbons about 1cm (½in) wide and place in a wide bowl.
- In a small bowl, mix together the mayonnaise, yogurt, vinegar, anchovies and capers.
- Stir the mayonnaise mixture gently into the lettuce and transfer to a serving bowl.
- Place the olives on the top and sprinkle with the Parmesan and black pepper.

Celeriac remoulade with smoked trout

164 calories

Think of this as a tangy celeriac coleslaw.

Serves 1   Preparation time: 15 minutes

¼ small celeriac, about 150g (5oz) peeled weight (27 cals)

50g (1¾oz) rocket (arugula) (13 cals)

2 tbsp extra-light mayonnaise (24 cals)

1 tbsp capers, chopped (2 cals)

juice ½ lemon (2 cals)

1 gherkin or 2 cornichons, chopped (4 cals)

salt and freshly ground black pepper

60g (2¼oz) smoked trout, cut into large slices (92 cals)

lemon wedge, to serve

- Peel the celeriac and coarsely grate. Combine the grated celeriac with the rocket (arugula).
- In a small bowl, mix together the mayonnaise, capers, lemon juice and chopped gherkin. Season with salt and pepper.
- Pour the dressing over the celeriac and mix until the celeriac and rocket are both covered.
- Arrange the smoked trout over the top and serve with a lemon wedge.

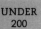
Japanese-style sake prawn salad

140 calories

A very healthy Japanese-style salad, it can be made with either fresh or frozen prawns.

Serves 2   Preparation time: 4 minutes   Cook time: 5–8 minutes

Quick & easy

2 tbsp sake (38 cals)
pinch of salt
juice of 1 lime (3 cals)
½ tsp wasabi powder
2 tsp olive oil (54 cals)
1 garlic clove, peeled and crushed (3 cals)
2 spring onions (scallions), trimmed and sliced (9 cals)
200g (7oz) raw king prawns (king or jumbo shrimp), fresh or frozen, peeled and deveined (152 cals)
150g (5oz) bagged young leaf salad, to serve (21 cals)

- In a small bowl, mix together 2 tablespoons water, the sake, salt, lime juice and wasabi powder.
- Heat the oil in a wide frying pan (skillet) over a high heat. When hot, add the garlic and spring onions (scallions) and fry lightly for 1–2 minutes. Tip in the prawns (shrimp) and cook for about 2 minutes (fresh) or 4 minutes (frozen), until they just start to turn pink.
- Tip in the sake mixture and bring up to a vigorous simmer. Cook for 2 minutes, stirring occasionally.
- When the prawns are cooked, serve on a bed of the salad with a little of the sauce from the pan drizzled over.

Garlicky king prawns

134 calories

This has to be one of my favourite quick suppers ever! Fresh raw prawns are used for this dish. If you want to use frozen prawns, defrost on a paper towel for two hours before use.

Serves 2   Preparation time: 5 minutes   Cook time: 4 minutes

Quick & easy

200g (7oz) raw king prawns (king or jumbo shrimp), peeled and deveined (152 cals)
salt and freshly ground black pepper
1 tsp olive oil (27 cals)
3 garlic cloves, peeled and crushed (9 cals)
10g (2 tsp) butter (74 cals)
small handful of flat-leaf (Italian) parsley (10g/⅓oz), chopped (3 cals)
juice of ½ lemon (2 cals)

- Dry the prawns (shrimp) by patting them with kitchen paper (paper towels) all over, then season with salt and pepper.
- Heat the oil in a wide frying pan (skillet) over a high heat. When the oil is very hot, add the prawns and stir-fry for 2 minutes. Add the garlic and fry for 1 more minute. Reduce the heat and stir in the butter. Cook for 1 more minute, or until the prawns are cooked through.
- Turn off the heat and stir in the parsley and lemon juice. Serve immediately.

Saffron 'rice' cauliflower

61 calories

As we all know, one of the big difficulties when dieting is to find filling, carb-like plate fillers that don't have too many calories. A rice alternative made with finely chopped cauliflower is one of my easy swaps for a fast day. This spicy dish goes superbly well with any of the curries in this book and really hits the spot.

If you want a simpler alternative, try putting the chopped cauliflower in a microwaveable dish. Add 2 tablespoons water, salt and pepper and cover, then microwave on high for 6 minutes.

Serves 2   Preparation time: 5 minutes   Cook time: 15 minutes

Vegetarian

½ small cauliflower (200g/7oz), cut into small florets (68 cals)
1 tsp sunflower oil (27 cals)
½ onion, peeled and finely chopped (27 cals)
1 cardamom pod
½ tsp turmeric
2 saffron strands
salt and freshly ground black pepper

- Put the cauliflower florets into a food processor and blitz until the cauliflower becomes small grains.
- Heat the oil in a wide lidded pan over a medium heat. Add the onion and fry for 5 minutes until tender and turning crisp at the edges.
- Break the cardamom pod open by pressing firmly with the flat side of a knife.
- Reduce the heat and add the cardamom, turmeric, saffron and salt and pepper to the pan, then stir in. Add the cauliflower and stir until coated in the onion and spice mixture.
- Add 3 tablespoons water, put the lid on and cook for 6–8 minutes until the cauliflower is tender.

Oven-baked vegetable fritters

149 calories

Serves 2   Preparation time: 5 minutes   Cook time: 1 hour

Vegetarian

2 small sweet potatoes, about 200g (7oz) in total (174 cals)
½ red onion, peeled and finely diced (27 cals)
½ green (bell) pepper, deseeded and finely diced (12 cals)
1 tsp olive oil (27 cals)
1 tsp cornflour (cornstarch), dissolved in a little cold water (18 cals)
1 spring onion (scallion), cut into fine rings (5 cals)
150g (scant 1 cup) cooked sweetcorn (drained weight) (34 cals)
salt and freshly ground black pepper
salad and lemon wedges, to serve

- Preheat the oven to 200°C/180°C fan/400°F/Gas mark 6 and line a baking tray with baking parchment or a silicone sheet.
- Prick the sweet potatoes all over with a fork and bake in the oven for 30–45 minutes, depending on size.
- Place the onion, pepper and oil in a small microwaveable bowl and cover with clingfilm (plastic wrap). Cook on high in the microwave for 2 minutes, then rest, covered, for a further 2 minutes.
- Cut the cooked sweet potato in half and squeeze the cooked sweet potato flesh out into a bowl. Stir in the cornflour (cornstarch). Add the cooked onion and pepper, spring onion (scallion) and sweetcorn, then season generously with salt and pepper and mix thoroughly.
- Using your hands, form the potato mixture into 4 balls, then place on the lined baking tray and press down gently with the palm of your hand to make a patty.
- Bake in the oven for about 15 minutes until just starting to brown on top.
- Serve with green salad and a wedge of lemon on the side.

Courgette ribbons with tomato and chorizo sauce

158 calories

Use thinly sliced courgette as an alternative to pasta in this dish.

Serves 1   Preparation time: 10 minutes   Cook time: 15 minutes

Quick & easy

1 large or 2 small courgettes, trimmed (45 cals)
20g (¾oz) chorizo, thinly sliced (58 cals)
1 garlic clove, peeled and thinly sliced (3 cals)
1 tbsp tomato purée (paste) (30 cals)
10 ripe cherry tomatoes, halved (22 cals)

- Use a vegetable peeler or mandoline to cut the courgette into ribbons. Discard the first slice as it will be mainly skin. If using the vegetable peeler, make slices until you hit the seeds, then rotate and peel again.
- Heat a frying pan (skillet) over a medium heat. When hot, toss in the chorizo and allow to sizzle and brown. Remove the chorizo from the pan and set aside, leaving the oil that has been released from the chorizo in the pan.
- Add the garlic and fry until golden. Next, add the tomato purée (paste) and stir-fry for 30 seconds before tossing in the courgettes. Stir-fry for another 1–2 minutes.
- Finally, add the tomatoes, reduce the heat and cook slowly for about 10 minutes. Serve sprinkled with the reserved chorizo.

Quick tomato and mangetout curry

144 calories

This low-calorie, vegetarian curry can be served on its own as a curry soup, with cauliflower 'rice' (see page 48) or with basmati rice. If serving with rice, allow 140 calories for a 40g (scant ¼ cup) (dry weight) portion.

Serves 2   Preparation time: 10 minutes   Cook time: 25 minutes

Vegetarian, quick & easy, freezer-friendly

1 tbsp olive oil (99 cals)

1 medium onion, peeled and chopped (54 cals)

pinch of salt

2 garlic cloves, peeled and finely sliced (6 cals)

1 tsp turmeric

1 tsp chilli powder

1 tsp garam masala

½ tsp English mustard (6 cals)

500g (1lb 2oz) cherry tomatoes (about 40), halved (90 cals)

100g (3½oz) mangetout (snow peas) (32 cals)

- Heat the oil in a large lidded saucepan over a low-medium heat. Add the onion and salt and fry gently for 5 minutes, stirring occasionally.
- Stir in the garlic and fry for another 2 minutes.
- Stir in the spices and mustard and then tip in the tomatoes. Put the lid on the pan and cook gently for 10–15 minutes or until the tomatoes break apart when pressed with the back of the spoon. Remove the lid and if necessary pick out any loose tomato skins.
- When the tomatoes are nearly cooked, remove the lid and add the mangetout (snow peas). Simmer gently for 2–3 minutes, then serve.

Cajun fried chicken

193 calories (including 9 cals from spice mix)

The spice mix here is enough to make 6–8 portions, so make a batch
and store the rest of the spices in an airtight container or jar.

Serves 1   Preparation time: 5 minutes   Cook time: 6–8 minutes

Quick & easy

1 x 150g (5oz) skinless chicken breast (159 cals)

1 tsp sunflower oil (27 cals)

For the spice mix (69 cals in total):

5 tsp ground cumin

2 heaped tsp smoked paprika (28 cals)

2 heaped tsp hot paprika (28 cals)

2 tsp dried thyme (3 cals)

2 tsp dried oregano (6 cals)

½ tsp cayenne pepper (2 cals)

1 tsp salt

- For the spice mix, mix together the spices and salt and set aside.
- Cut the chicken into 4–5 strips. Sprinkle 2 teaspoons of the spice
  mix over and use your hands to toss through.
- Heat the oil in a shallow frying pan (skillet) over a medium-high
  heat. When hot, toss in the chicken and cook for 3–4 minutes on
  each side, until golden and cooked through. Serve.

Garlic grilled chicken

187 calories

This dish is marinated in a milky sauce, giving it a wonderful succulence. I have given a recommended marinating time of 30 minutes but it is even better if left for an hour or even overnight in the fridge.

Serves 2   Preparation time: 7 minutes, plus chilling
Cook time: 20 minutes

150ml (⅔ cup) skimmed (skim) milk (48 cals)
juice of ½ lemon (2 cals)
2 garlic cloves, peeled and crushed (6 cals)
salt and freshly ground black pepper
2 × 150g (5oz) skinless chicken breasts (318 cals)

- Combine the skimmed milk and lemon juice in a jug (pitcher) and leave to stand for 5 minutes. During this time the milk will curdle. Stir in the garlic and salt and pepper.
- Lightly score the chicken breasts, then place in a wide bowl and pour the milk over. Turn the chicken in the sauce to make sure it is fully covered. Cover the bowl with clingfilm (plastic wrap), then chill for at least 30 minutes.
- When you are ready to cook the chicken, heat the grill (broiler) to a medium-high setting. Remove the chicken from the marinade and place on a grill pan. When the grill has reached the correct temperature, grill (broil) the chicken for 7–10 minutes on each side until cooked through.

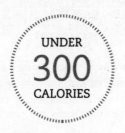

UNDER
300
CALORIES

Power up breakfast

219 calories

This is one of my favourite breakfasts on any day of the week. It's easier than porridge yet just as filling. Some people might prefer to prepare the night before and rest overnight. I don't bother as I prefer it with a bit of crunch.

Serves 1   Preparation time: 2 minutes

Quick & easy

30g (⅓ cup) porridge (rolled) oats (107 cals)

10g (small handful) oat granola (42 cals)

150ml (⅔ cup) skimmed (skim) milk (48 cals)

1 tbsp low-fat yogurt (22 cals)

- Simply combine all the ingredients together and stir.

Baked eggs with ham and tomato

251 calories

This is a mini potted breakfast.

Serves 1   Preparation time: 5 minutes   Cook time: 15 minutes

Quick & easy

½ leek, trimmed and thinly sliced (13 cals)
½ tsp olive oil (14 cals)
1 slice ham, chopped (41 cals)
1 large egg (91 cals)
2 slices tomato (9 cals)
20g (scant ¼ cup) Cheddar cheese, grated (83 cals)

- Preheat the oven to 180°C/160°C fan/350°F/Gas mark 4.
- Place the leek and oil in a small microwaveable dish. Cover with clingfilm (plastic wrap) and microwave on high for 4 minutes. Leave to rest, still covered, for a further 2 minutes.
- Place the leek at the bottom of a ramekin and top with the ham.
- Pour in the egg, then top with the tomato slices and sprinkle with the cheese.
- Bake in the oven for 10 minutes or until the egg is set and the top is turning brown.

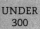
Smoked fish chowder

251 calories

This is low-fat comfort food and is perfect for warming you up on a wet spring day.

Serves 4   Preparation time: 5 minutes   Cook time: 35 minutes

Extra-filling, quick & easy, freezer-friendly

10 black peppercorns
1 bay leaf
400g (14oz) skinless smoked haddock or cod (324 cals)
500ml (generous 2 cups) skimmed (skim) milk (160 cals)
500ml (generous 2 cups) fish or vegetable stock (fresh or made with 1 cube) (35 cals)
1 tsp olive oil (27 cals)
4 leeks, trimmed and cut into thin rings (106 cals)
½ tsp cumin seeds
500g (1lb 2 oz) new potatoes, skin on, quartered (350 cals)

- Place the peppercorns, bay leaf and fish in a saucepan. Pour in the milk and stock and bring to a gentle simmer. Continue to simmer gently until just cooked through, about 6–8 minutes. Remove the fish from the pan and set aside, reserving the cooking liquid.
- Meanwhile in a wide lidded frying pan (skillet), heat the oil over a low heat and stir in the leeks. Put the lid on and soften the leeks for 10 minutes.
- Remove the lid from the leeks and turn up the heat. Add the cumin seeds and fry until they start to sizzle and pop, then stir in the potatoes. Pour in the poaching liquid from the fish and bring to the boil. Reduce the heat and simmer for 15–20 minutes until the potatoes are tender.
- Turn off the heat. Break the fish apart gently with your fingers and add to the soup. Heat gently for 1–2 minutes before serving.

Quick tomato haddock

225 calories

This dish is an easy way to liven up any white fish.

Serves 1   Preparation time: 10 minutes   Cook time: 25 minutes

Quick & easy

1 tsp olive oil (27 cals)

½ onion, peeled and finely diced (27 cals)

1 tbsp tomato purée (paste) (30 cals)

2 medium tomatoes, diced (28 cals)

½ tsp brown sugar (9 cals)

1 fresh oregano sprig (optional)

1 tsp soy sauce (2 cals)

1 skinless haddock fillet, about 125g (4oz)

(101 cals)

- In a small lidded saucepan, heat the oil over a low-medium heat. Add the onion and fry lightly for 5 minutes, until tinged with brown. Stir in the tomato purée (paste) and fry for 1 more minute.
- Add 2 tablespoons water, tomatoes, sugar, oregano and soy sauce. Reduce the heat to low, put the lid on and simmer for 5 minutes.
- Lower the fish carefully into the pan and spoon the sauce over so that it is fully covered. Put the lid back on the pan and gently cook for about 10 minutes until the fish is cooked and flakes easily.

Purple sprouting broccoli with creamy caper sauce

230 calories

Serves 1   Preparation time: 5 minutes   Cook time: 20 minutes

Vegetarian, quick & easy

1 tsp olive oil (27 cals)
1 shallot, peeled and finely chopped (6 cals)
1 garlic clove, peeled and finely chopped (3 cals)
1 tbsp capers, drained (2 cals)
1 medium tomato, finely chopped (14 cals)
100ml (scant ½ cup) vegetable stock (fresh or made with ¼ cube) (9 cals)
1 tbsp double (heavy) cream (135 cals)
salt
100g (3½oz) purple sprouting (or Tenderstem) broccoli, trimmed (34 cals)

- Heat the oil in a frying pan (skillet), add the shallot and gently fry until softened. Add the garlic and cook for 1 minute.
- Add the capers, tomato and stock. Bring to the boil, then reduce the heat and simmer gently for 10 minutes. Turn off the heat. If preferred you can blend the sauce until smooth at this stage. Stir in the cream.
- Meanwhile, bring a saucepan of lightly salted water to the boil and plunge in the broccoli. Cook for 4–6 minutes until just tender.
- Arrange the broccoli on a plate and pour the sauce over.

Patatas bravas

248 calories

This is my take on the classic Spanish dish.

Serves 1   Preparation time: 10 minutes   Cook time: 40 minutes

Quick & easy

180g (6½oz) new potatoes (about 4 small),
with skin on (126 cals)

salt and freshly ground black pepper

1 tsp olive oil (27 cals)

1 shallot, peeled and diced (6 cals)

1 garlic clove, peeled and sliced (3 cals)

1 red chilli, finely chopped (3 cals)

1 tbsp tomato purée (paste) (30 cals)

pinch of sugar

¼ tsp smoked paprika (2 cals)

1 tsp sunflower oil (27 cals)

10 ripe cherry tomatoes, halved (22 cals)

1 tbsp red wine vinegar (2 cals)

- Quarter the new potatoes and place in a saucepan of cold salted water. Bring the pan to the boil and cook until tender. This will take 12–15 minutes from cold. When cooked, drain the potatoes and lay on kitchen paper (paper towels) to cool and dry.
- Heat the olive oil in a frying pan (skillet) over a medium heat. Add the shallot and cook for 5 minutes before adding the garlic and red chilli and frying for another 2 minutes.

continued

- Stir in the tomato purée (paste), a pinch of salt, the sugar and paprika and fry for 1 minute before tossing in the tomatoes and vinegar. Cook gently for 10–15 minutes until thick. If it starts to stick to the pan add a little water to loosen the sauce.

- When the potatoes are cool, heat the sunflower oil in a wide pan over a high heat. When hot, add the potatoes and stir once. Leave to fry until golden on one side, do not stir, this will take about 3 minutes. Turn the potatoes and fry for a further 3 minutes until crispy and brown all over.

- Loosely stir the potatoes into the sauce and serve immediately with a generous sprinkling of black pepper.

Warming leek 'pasta' with olives

233 calories

Hearty, warming and filling, what's not to like?

Serves 1   Preparation time: 5 minutes   Cook time: 12 minutes

Vegetarian, quick & easy

1 tsp olive oil (27 cals)
2 leeks, trimmed and cut into 1cm (½in) wide slices (52 cals)
zest of 1 lemon
juice of ½ lemon (2 cals)
1 tsp extra virgin olive oil (27 cals)
salt and freshly ground black pepper
10g (2 tbsp) Parmesan, fresh grated (83 cals)
50g (1¾oz) watercress or baby spinach leaves (11 cals)
6 black olives, pitted (31 cals)

- In a wide lidded pan, heat the olive oil over a medium-high heat. When hot, add the leeks and stir-fry for 2 minutes. Reduce the heat, add about 2 tablespoons water and put the lid on. Steam until tender, about 10 minutes.
- Combine the lemon zest, lemon juice, extra virgin olive oil, salt and pepper and half the Parmesan in a small bowl.
- Stir the watercress, olives and lemon dressing through the leek pasta.
- Transfer to a serving bowl and sprinkle on the remaining Parmesan. Season generously with salt and pepper and serve.

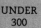

Asian-style stir-fried beef and mushrooms

267 calories

I use pre-prepared stir-fry veg here for simplicity. If you want to use fresh own veg, try a combination of beansprouts, cabbage, carrot and onion. The overnight marinating is not essential – it just adds depth of flavour and makes the beef deliciously tender.

Serves 2   Preparation time: 10 minutes, plus marinating
Cook time: 7 minutes

2 tbsp dark soy sauce (9 cals)
juice of 1 lime (4 cals)
1 tsp sesame oil (30 cals)
½ tsp chilli (red pepper) flakes
200g (7oz) extra lean beef steak, cut into slivers (246 cals)
2 tsp sunflower oil (54 cals)
250g (9oz) mushrooms, sliced (32 cals)
1 × 300g (11oz) pack mixed vegetable stir-fry (158 cals)

- In a wide dish, mix together the soy sauce, lime juice, sesame oil and chilli flakes. Add the steak, turning to make sure all the pieces are fully covered. Cover the dish with clingfilm (plastic wrap) and leave to marinate – the longer the better, anything from 30 minutes to overnight.
- Heat the sunflower oil in a wok or wide frying pan (skillet) to a high temperature. Lift the beef from the marinade (setting the marinade aside for later) and stir-fry for 2 minutes until browned. Remove the meat from the wok and set aside.
- With the heat still on high, add the mushrooms and stir-fry for 2 minutes, then add the mixed veg and stir-fry for 1 more minute. Reduce the heat a little and return the beef to the pan. Pour over the rest of the marinade and toss everything together for 2 minutes until piping hot.

Grilled lamb in fresh parsley and mint sauce

241 calories

You really need some fresh parsley and mint for this sauce but it is well worth it. Prepare the sauce first, it works better if the flavours are left to combine for a few minutes. The sauce keeps well in the fridge for a few days.

Serves 2   Preparation time: 10 minutes   Cook time: 15 minutes

1 garlic clove, peeled (4 cals)
salt and freshly ground black pepper
2 fresh mint leaves
large bunch of flat-leaf (Italian) parsley (10g/⅓oz) (3 cals)
juice of 1 lemon (3 cals)
2 tbsp extra virgin olive oil (198 cals)
2 × 90g (3¼oz) lean lamb leg steaks (275 cals)

- Place the garlic, a little salt, the herbs and lemon juice in a blender and process until they form a paste. If you don't have a blender, you can chop the ingredients finely instead. Gradually pour in the olive oil, blending until it forms a smooth emulsified sauce. Transfer the sauce to a wide dish that is big enough to hold the lamb.

- Preheat the grill (broiler) to medium-high. Season the lamb and place under the grill. Cook for 5–8 minutes on each side, depending on how you like your lamb. It should be seared on the outside and if you like it a little pink, you should make sure the inside gets properly hot – 145°C/293°F on a meat thermometer.

- Transfer the lamb to the serving dish and scoop up the sauce over the top. Leave to rest in the sauce for a few minutes before serving.

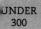

Vietnamese yellow curry

251 calories

This curry has a beautiful colour and aroma. I like to serve this on a bed of lightly steamed spring greens or spinach. I have used chicken breast here, but substituting the cheaper chicken thighs gives it a greater depth of flavour.

Serves 2   Preparation time: 10 minutes   Cook time: 2–5 hours

Freezer-friendly, slow cooking

2 tsp sunflower oil (54 cals)
6 spring onions (scallions), shredded (30 cals)
1 garlic clove, peeled and finely chopped (3 cals)
250g (9oz) skinless chicken breast, cut into rough cubes (265 cals)
1 tsp ground turmeric
½ tsp ground ginger
½ tsp ground cumin
½ stick lemongrass, finely chopped
1 green chilli, deseeded and finely chopped (1 cal)
½ can (200ml/generous ¾ cup) light coconut milk, shaken (146 cals)
handful of fresh coriander (cilantro) (10g/⅓oz), roughly chopped (optional) (2 cals)

- Preheat the oven to 140°C/120° fan/275°F/Gas mark 1.
- Heat the oil in a wide frying pan (skillet) over a medium–high heat. When hot, toss in the spring onions (scallions), garlic and chicken and fry for 3 minutes. Stir and turn the chicken halfway through cooking. Stir in the spices, lemongrass and chilli and cook for 1–2 minutes.

continued

- Transfer the chicken mixture to a small casserole dish or slow cooker. Pour the coconut milk over, making sure the chicken is covered. Top up with a little water if necessary.
- Cook covered in the oven for 2 hours OR in a slow cooker on low for 5 hours.

Slow-baked chicken rolls in tomato sauce

274 calories

This is a great one-pot dish where you just pop your ingredients in the casserole dish and leave it to cook slowly.

Serves 4   Preparation time: 5 minutes   Cook time: 3–6 hours

Freezer-friendly, slow cooking

100g (3½oz) sausagemeat (309 cals)

4 skinless, boneless chicken thighs, about 360g (392 cals)

1 onion, peeled and chopped (654 cals)

2 garlic cloves, peeled and finely chopped (6 cals)

1 red (bell) pepper, deseeded and roughly chopped (45 cals)

1 green (bell) pepper, deseeded and roughly chopped (24 cals)

1 × 400g (14oz) can butter (lima) beans, rinsed and drained (182 cals)

1 × 400g (14oz) can chopped tomatoes (64 cals)

½ chicken stock (bouillon) cube (18 cals)

1 tsp dried oregano (3 cals)

continued

- Preheat the oven to 140°C/120°C fan/275°F/Gas mark 1 if using the oven.

- Divide the sausagemeat into roughly 4 equal portions. Open up the chicken thighs and lay them flat. Place the portion of sausagemeat in the middle of the chicken and pull up the sides so that the meat is enclosed in a tight roll. If you wish to make a neater parcel you can hold the two ends of the chicken together with a cocktail stick (toothpick). Turn the chicken roll over so that the join is on the bottom.

- Use a large casserole dish or slow cooker dish. Layer the onion, garlic and peppers at the base of the dish, then add the butter (lima) beans. Place the stuffed chicken thighs on top and pour on the chopped tomatoes. Crunch up the stock (bouillon) cube in your fingers and sprinkle over the top. Add the oregano. Finally, top up with 300ml (1¼ cups) water until the chicken is generously covered.

- Cook in the oven for 3 hours. Alternatively, cook in the slow cooker for at least 6 hours.

Blueberry fool

212 calories

A lovely easy treat, this pudding can be kept, covered, in the fridge for up to 24 hours.

Serves 4   Preparation time: 10 minutes, plus chilling

500g (3⅓ cups) blueberries, washed (285 cals)
450ml (2 cups) low-fat plain yogurt (252 cals)
4 tbsp light crème fraîche (227 cals)
zest from 2 lemons (4 cals)
½ tsp ground cinnamon
2 tsp icing (confectioners') sugar (79 cals)

- Set aside 16 blueberries for the top of the fools.
- Place the rest of the blueberries in a food processor or blender and process until smooth. If you prefer you can pass the blueberries through a sieve (strainer) at this stage to remove the skins.
- Mix the yogurt, crème fraîche, lemon zest, cinnamon and icing (confectioners') sugar in a bowl. Fold the blueberry sauce through the yogurt and transfer to 4 serving dishes or goblets.
- Chill for at least 30 minutes.
- Top with 4 reserved blueberries per pudding before serving.

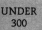

Baked banana with dark chocolate

221 calories

This is a classic I remember from my days as a Brownie!

Serves 1   Preparation time: 5 minutes   Cook time: 10 minutes

1 medium banana, unpeeled (119 cals)

20g (¾oz/6 squares) good-quality dark chocolate,
roughly chopped (102 cals)

- Preheat the oven to 190°C/170°C fan/375°F/Gas mark 5.
- Cut a slit along the top length of the banana, cutting slightly into the flesh but making sure it is attached at both ends.
- Push the chocolate into the slit and cover with the skin.
- Wrap the banana loosely in foil.
- Place the banana in the oven with the slit side uppermost and bake for 10 minutes until the skin is black and the chocolate has melted.

Crème de menthe pudding with chocolate crunch

270 calories

A quick and 'cheaty' pudding, feel free to leave out the green food colouring if you don't want it too green.

Serves 2   Preparation time: 5 minutes   Cook time: 5 minutes

1 level tbsp cornflour (cornstarch) (53 cals)
2 tbsp caster (superfine) sugar (158 cals)
300ml (1¼ cups) skimmed (skim) milk (96 cals)
1 tbsp light soft cheese (55 cals)
2 tbsp Crème de menthe (111 cals)
2 drops green food colouring
1 bourbon biscuit (cookie) (67 cals)

- Place the cornflour (cornstarch) and sugar in a non-stick saucepan. Add a small amount of milk and stir until you have a smooth paste with no lumps. Add a little more milk and stir again. Pour in the rest of the milk and make sure the paste is fully combined.
- Turn the heat to high. Start stirring with a balloon whisk and continue to whisk gently as the milk heats up and starts to bubble. When the sauce is of a thick consistency turn off the heat but continue to whisk for another minute as the sauce cools.
- Mix in the soft cheese first then the Crème de menthe and food colouring. When totally smooth and combined, transfer the mixture to 2 ramekins. Crumble over the bourbon biscuits and serve immediately.

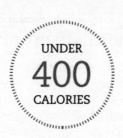

UNDER
400
CALORIES

Paprika chicken salad

300 calories

One of my favourite easy salads, the chicken is very tender when quick fried in this way.

Serves 1   Preparation time: 5 minutes   Cook time: 10 minutes

Quick & easy

1 × 150g (5oz) skinless chicken breast, cut into 4–5 slices (159 cals)
½ level tbsp plain (all-purpose) flour (34 cals)
salt and freshly ground black pepper
½ tsp paprika (3 cals)
1 tsp olive oil (27 cals)
100g (3½oz) bag baby leaf salad (21 cals)
100g (3½oz) cucumber (about 5cm/2in piece), roughly chopped (10 cals)
10 cherry tomatoes, halved (22 cals)
1 tbsp low-fat plain yogurt (22 cals)
¼ tsp paprika (2 cals)

continued

- Place the chicken in a bowl and sprinkle on the flour, salt and pepper and ½ teaspoon paprika. Use your hands to toss the chicken in the flour and make sure it is evenly covered.
- Heat the oil in a frying pan (skillet) over a medium heat. When hot, add the chicken and fry for about 4 minutes on each side, depending on thickness.
- Meanwhile, prepare all your salad ingredients and place in a serving bowl. Combine the yogurt and ¼ teaspoon paprika in a small cup.
- Place the just cooked chicken on top of the salad and drizzle the yogurt dressing over.

Spring chicken stew

365 calories

This is a pleasing and quick chicken stew.

Serves 2   Preparation time: 15 minutes   Cook time: 40–50 minutes

Freezer-friendly

50g (¼ cup) chopped streaky bacon or lardons (138 cals)
2 skinless, boneless chicken thighs, about 360g (12oz) (392 cals)
½ leek, trimmed and roughly chopped (13 cals)
1 celery stick, finely sliced (2 cals)
2 garlic cloves, peeled and finely sliced (6 cals)
1 tsp mixed dried herbs (3 g/⅛ oz) (8 cals)
200ml (generous ¾ cup) dry (hard) cider (72 cals)
80g (¾ cup) frozen peas (53 cals)
1 tbsp Dijon mustard (28 cals)
salt and freshly ground black pepper
1 Little Gem (Boston) lettuce, roughly shredded (17 cals)
fresh tarragon (optional)

continued

- Heat the chopped bacon or lardons in a heavy-based lidded saucepan, cooking them until they brown all over. Remove them from the pan with a slotted spoon and set aside. Add the chicken thighs and cook on the first side for about 5 minutes over a medium heat.
- Turn the chicken over and add the leek, celery, garlic and dried herbs. Give everything a stir and let it continue to cook for a further 5 minutes. Return the chopped bacon or lardons to the pan.
- Pour in the cider and add the peas. Bring to the boil, then reduce the heat, put the lid on and cook for 20–30 minutes until the chicken is cooked through.
- Remove the lid, stir in the mustard and season with salt and pepper. Finally, toss the lettuce and tarragon over the chicken and let it wilt into the sauce for about 2 minutes.
- Serve immediately.

Grilled lamb with tangy lemon couscous

314 calories

A lovely complete meal that can safely be fed to non-dieting friends without complaint!

Serves 2   Preparation time: 10 minutes   Cook time: 35 minutes

Quick & easy

1 tsp olive oil (27 cals)
1 garlic clove, peeled and finely sliced (3 cals)
100g (½ cup) couscous (dried weight) (227 cals)
250ml (generous 1 cup) hot chicken stock (made with ½ cube) (17 cals)
2 × 90g (3¼oz) lean lamb leg steaks (337 cals)

continued

salt and freshly ground black pepper
zest and juice of 1 lemon (4 cals)
50g (1¾oz) rocket (arugula) (13 cals)

- Heat the oil in a medium lidded saucepan over a medium heat. Add the garlic and fry for about 2 minutes or until golden, then stir in the couscous. Fry the couscous for 1–2 minutes, stirring constantly. Turn the heat off.

- Add the hot stock to the couscous and stir gently. Put the lid on the pan and leave the couscous to 'cook' for about 15 minutes. When cooked all the liquid will have been absorbed and the couscous will be tender with just a little bite.

- While the couscous is cooking, heat the grill (broiler) to a medium-high setting.

- Season the lamb with salt and pepper and place under the hot grill. The cooking time will depend on thickness and desired degree of doneness. Anything from 5–8 minutes on each side. If you have a meat thermometer the internal temp should reach 145°C/293°F.

- Set the lamb aside and cover for 5 minutes. Resting makes the meat more tender.

- When both the lamb and couscous are done, stir the lemon zest and juice of half the lemon into the couscous, then stir in the rocket (arugula).

- Serve with the lamb resting on top of the couscous and squeezing on a little of the remaining lemon juice.

Spicy lamb keema

316 calories

This is quick and easy to rustle up after work.

Serves 4   Preparation time: 10 minutes, plus marinating

Cook time: 20 minutes

Freezer-friendly

4 tbsp mirin (137 cals)
1 tbsp honey (86 cals)
1 tbsp miso paste (41 cals)
1 tbsp mild chilli powder
2 tbsp dark soy sauce (13 cals)
400g (14oz) lean minced (ground) lamb (784 cals)
1 tsp vegetable oil (27 cals)
8 spring onions (scallions), chopped (40 cals)
200g (1¾ cups) peas, fresh or frozen (132 cals)
handful of fresh coriander (cilantro) (10g/⅓oz), chopped (2 cals)

- Mix together the mirin, honey, miso paste, chilli powder and soy sauce.
- Break the lamb apart with your fingers and put into a large bowl. Pour the sauce over and mix together. Leave to marinate for 5–10 minutes.
- Heat the oil in a large frying pan (skillet) over a medium-high heat. When hot, toss in the spring onions (scallions) and stir-fry for 2 minutes.
- Tip any extra sauce out of the lamb and set aside for later. Add the lamb to the pan and stir-fry until brown all over. Stir in the peas.

continued

- Add 200ml (generous ¾ cup) water, bring up to a simmer then reduce the heat to low. Add any remaining sauce from the meat and cook for 15 minutes.
- Stir in the chopped coriander before serving.

Slow-cooked stuffed cabbage rolls

343 calories

This is a classic Czech dish. The cabbage rolls freeze very well – either before or after cooking.

Serves 6   Preparation time: 30 minutes   Cook time: 2¼ hours

Freezer-friendly, slow cooking

1 large green cabbage, about 1kg/2¼lb (270 cals)
salt and freshly ground black pepper
1 medium onion, peeled and finely chopped (54 cals)
1 tsp olive oil (27 cals)
500g (1lb 2oz) lean minced (ground) beef (870 cals)
250g (9oz) lean minced (ground) pork (410 cals)
1 × 400g (14oz) can cooked Puy lentils, rinsed and drained (278 cals)
1 large egg (91 cals)
1 heaped tsp paprika (14 cals)
300ml (1¼ cups) tomato juice (42 cals)

- Remove the core from the cabbage with a sharp knife.
- Place the whole head of cabbage in a large saucepan of boiling salted water. Put the lid on and cook for 3 minutes.
- Remove the cabbage from the pan and leave to cool slightly. Pull off the individual outer leaves. You will need about 18 leaves.

continued

- Preheat the oven to 170°C/150°C fan/325°F/Gas mark 3.
- Using scissors or a sharp knife, cut away the thick centre stem of each leaf, being careful not to cut all the way through.
- Chop the remaining cabbage and place it at the base of a large casserole dish.
- Fry the onion slowly in the oil for 10 minutes. Leave to cool.
- Break apart the minced (ground) beef and pork into a large bowl. Add the lentils, egg, paprika and onion and season generously with salt and pepper. Mix all the ingredients together with your hands until fully combined.
- Place a generous tablespoon of filling on a cabbage leaf. Lift the nearside of the cabbage over the meat and roll away from you to encase it. Flip the sides of the leaf into the middle and roll away from you again to create a neat packet. Place on top of the chopped cabbage in the casserole dish.
- Repeat with the rest of the cabbage leaves, making layers of rolls in the casserole dish.
- Pour the tomato juice over the rolls in the casserole dish and bring to the boil on the hob.
- Put the lid on and cook in the oven for 2 hours. Alternatively, cook in a slow cooker for 6–8 hours.

Creamy purple sprouting broccoli with Parma ham

337 calories

Serves 1   Preparation time: 5 minutes   Cook time: 25 minutes

180g (6½oz) new potatoes (about 4 small),
with skin on (126 cals)

salt and freshly ground black pepper

75ml (⅓ cup) light crème fraîche (122 cals)

1 frond fresh dill, finely chopped

100g (3½oz) purple sprouting (or Tenderstem) broccoli,
trimmed (35 cals)

2 slices Parma ham (prosciutto), cut into pieces (54 cals)

- For the potatoes, bring a large pan of salted water to the boil. Add the potatoes and cook for 20 minutes or until tender. Drain the potatoes and cut into quarters.
- Mix the crème fraîche, dill and a little salt and pepper together in a large heatproof bowl. Gently toss the hot potatoes in the dressing.
- Meanwhile, bring another saucepan of lightly salted water to the boil and plunge in the broccoli. Cook for 4–6 minutes until just tender.
- Lightly combine the broccoli with the potatoes, being careful not to break up the spears.
- Arrange the pieces of Parma ham (prosciutto) over the potatoes and broccoli and serve immediately.

SUMMER

SUMMER RECIPES

Under 200 calories

Healthy blueberry bran muffins
Classic smoked salmon with scrambled eggs
Fresh tomato and chilli soup
Vietnamese king prawns and sugar snaps
Roasted aubergine with spicy yogurt dressing
Harissa spiced chickpeas on green beans
Smoky BBQ chicken
Chilled strawberries and Cointreau
Honey glazed pineapple
Vanilla ice cream soda
Raspberry sorbet
Peach Melba

Under 300 calories

Classic Greek salad

Tangy bulgur wheat and broad bean salad

Italian courgette and tomato salad

Avocado and bacon salad

Chicken salad with lemon pepper dressing

Courgette 'pizza' bites

Asparagus pile up

Courgette and feta fritters

Oven-baked sweet potato wedges with real aïoli

Super easy crushed chickpeas with Boursin

Spicy bean burgers

Caribbean casserole

Lime and chilli prawns with salsa

Fiery coconut crab cakes

Seared scallops with garlicky potatoes

Olive chicken and broccoli

Parmesan chicken

Chicken 'burger' with Portobello bun

Lamb with quick Cumberland sauce

Banana pancakes

Under 400 calories

Creamy salmon salad

Lamb tagine

Fragrant chicken

Rainy day stew

LOOK THE BEST THAT
YOU POSSIBLY CAN

The joys of summer: everybody's favourite season. It is the time for easy salads and family barbecues.

It is also the time when it is considered the easiest to diet and lose weight. You don't need as much body fat to keep you warm so you no longer crave or eat as much carbohydrate. This means you are naturally slimmer. BUT it doesn't always work like that, it can be a dangerous season for dieters too. We all want to enjoy ourselves in summer – a cold beer, fish and chips and ice cream all round. In the summer holidays you might find yourself surrounded by children for six weeks, making diet days immeasurably harder.

So summer is the time to be extra careful on your diet days, and make them really work for you. The 'hunger' should be less than when it is cold. Be more lenient with yourself on your other days, and allow yourself some treats. I wouldn't want to deny anyone a glass of chilled white wine or an ice cream on the beach.

The trick for your diet days is to make the most of lean chicken and fish, served with large (and very low-calorie) salads. There are loads of options, and you will be surprised how much good food you can eat for 500 calories when you cut out the carbs. If you are feeding others, it should be easy to add potatoes or bread for the non-dieters and you shouldn't find it too hard to be virtuous.

My barbecue sauce in the Smoky BBQ chicken recipe (see page 93) is the most amazingly addictive topping, which works well with other meats besides chicken. If you are careful in your calories you can also allow yourself some of the fruity treats that the season provides. Try the Chilled strawberries and Cointreau (see page 94) for the ultimate in low-calorie puddings: it has only 99 calories per serving.

Menu plans for diet days

Use these planners to inspire your cooking on diet days. It's amazing how much good food you can eat for under 500–600 calories.

Just work out whether you want three small meals/breakfast and dinner/lunch and dinner on your diet days and choose the right planner for you. If you need more help working out which plan is right for you have a look at *What kind of dieter are you?* (see page 6).

Feel free to swap a recipe for another with a similar calorie content if necessary.

MENU PLANS FOR DIET DAYS: WOMEN (SUMMER)

WOMEN: 3 SMALL MEALS

	Breakfast	Lunch	Dinner	Cals
Day 1	Healthy blueberry bran muffin (page 87) 139 cals	Fresh tomato and chilli soup (page 89) 114 cals	Olive chicken and broccoli (page 113) 250 cals	503
Day 2	Healthy blueberry bran muffin (page 87) 139 cals	Roasted aubergine with spicy yogurt dressing (page 91) 110 cals	Seared scallops with garlicky potatoes (page 112) 252 cals	502

WOMEN: BREAKFAST AND DINNER

	Breakfast	Dinner	Cals
Day 1	Banana pancakes (page 117) 251 cals	Lamb with quick Cumberland sauce (page 116) 237 cals	488
Day 2	Classic smoked salmon with scrambled eggs (page 88) 182 cals	Rainy day stew (page 121) 312 cals	494

WOMEN: LUNCH AND DINNER

	Lunch	Dinner	Cals
Day 1	Classic Greek salad (page 98) 218 cals	Chicken 'burger' with Portobello bun (page 115) 281 cals	499
Day 2	Super easy crushed chickpeas with Boursin (page 107) 262 cals	Fiery coconut crab cakes (page 111) 233 cals	495

MENU PLANS FOR DIET DAYS: MEN (SUMMER)

MEN: 3 SMALL MEALS

	Breakfast	Lunch	Dinner	Cals
Day 1	Classic smoked salmon with scrambled eggs (page 88) 182 cals	Fresh tomato and chilli soup (page 89) 114 cals	Chicken salad with lemon pepper dressing (page 102) 294 cals	590
Day 2	1 egg, boiled (89) Slice of wholemeal (wholewheat) toast (110) 199 cals	Harissa spiced chickpeas on green beans (page 92) 184 cals	Smoky BBQ chicken (page 93) (197) 70g (2½oz) bag mixed leaf salad (16) 213 cals	596

MEN: BREAKFAST AND DINNER

	Breakfast	Dinner	Cals
Day 1	Banana pancakes (page 117) 251 cals	Fragrant chicken (page 120) 333 cals	584
Day 2	Classic smoked salmon with scrambled eggs (page 88) 182 cals	Lamb with quick Cumberland sauce (page 116) (237) 200g (7oz) new potatoes (4 small) (140) 100g (3½oz) broccoli (33) 410 cals	592

MEN: LUNCH AND DINNER

	Lunch	Dinner	Cals
Day 1	Courgette 'pizza' bites (page 103) 216 cals	Olive chicken and broccoli (page 113) (250) 200g (7oz) new potatoes (4 small) (140) 390 cals	606
Day 2	Classic Greek salad (page 98) 218 cals	Lamb tagine (page 119) (303) 40g (scant ¼ cup) couscous (91) 394 cals	612

SUMMER RECIPES

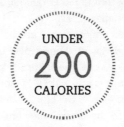

UNDER
200
CALORIES

Healthy blueberry bran muffins
139 calories

These make a healthy breakfast choice or an emergency mid-morning feast. You can also freeze the muffins in an airtight container and defrost them individually, although they are not quite as nice.

Makes 10 muffins   Preparation time: 10 minutes   Cook time: 20 minutes

Breakfast/snack, freezer-friendly

200ml (generous ¾ cup) skimmed milk (64 cals)

juice of ½ lemon (2 cals)

150g (generous 1 cup) plain (all-purpose) flour (512 cals)

100g (¾ cup) self-raising (self-rising) flour (330 cals)

1 tbsp oat bran (25 cals)

2 tsp baking powder (14 cals)

½ tsp bicarbonate of soda (baking soda)

pinch of salt

50g (¼ cup) muscovado (soft brown) sugar (181 cals)

1 tbsp runny honey (86 cals)

1 large egg (91 cals)

150g (1 cup) fresh blueberries (86 cals)   *continued*

- First combine the skimmed milk and lemon juice in a small bowl or jug (pitcher) and leave to rest for 5 minutes.
- Preheat the oven to 180°C/160°C fan/350°F/Gas mark 4. Line a muffin tray with 10 paper cases.
- Mix all the dry ingredients together in a large bowl.
- Whisk the honey and egg into the curdled milk with a fork.
- Pour the wet ingredients over the dry and mix until well combined. Don't worry if the mix is still a little lumpy, it is better to under rather than overmix. Fold in the blueberries.
- Spoon the batter into the paper cases and bake in the oven for about 20 minutes, until turning brown on the top.

Classic smoked salmon with scrambled eggs

182 calories

A classy breakfast to start your fast day right!

Serves 1   Preparation time: 2 minutes   Cook time: 3 minutes

Quick & easy

60g (2¼oz) smoked salmon (85 cals)
1 large egg (91 cals)
1 tbsp skimmed (skim) milk (5 cals)
squeeze of lemon juice (1 cal)
salt and freshly ground black pepper

- Arrange the smoked salmon on a serving plate.
- Crack the egg into a small non-stick saucepan and add the milk.
- Heat the egg gently while stirring continuously. Remove from the heat while the eggs are scrambled but still soft and place on the serving plate with the salmon.
- Squeeze the lemon juice over the salmon and season generously with salt and pepper. Serve immediately.

Fresh tomato and chilli soup

114 calories

If you have a glut of ripe or over-ripe tomatoes then this is the soup for you. As always I go for the easy option – no peeling or deseeding tomatoes here!

Serves 4 Preparation time: 10 minutes   Cook time: 35 minutes

Freezer-friendly

2 tsp olive oil (54 cals)

2 medium onions, peeled and cut into thin
half rings (108 cals)

2 red chillies, deseeded if preferred and diced (8 cals)

1 red (bell) pepper, chopped (54 cals)

salt and freshly ground black pepper

2 tbsp tomato purée (paste) (61 cals)

1kg (2¼lb) ripe tomatoes, very roughly chopped (170 cals)

- Heat the oil in a large lidded frying pan (skillet) over a medium heat. Add the onions, chillies and red (bell) pepper and fry for 3 minutes. Season generously with salt and pepper, then reduce the heat, put the lid on and cook slowly for 20 minutes, until tender.
- Increase the heat back and stir in the tomato purée (paste). Cook for 1 minute, then add the tomatoes, stir and put the lid back on. Reduce the heat to low and cook for a further 10 minutes.
- Stir and break up the some of the tomatoes with the back of the spoon. Remove any loose tomato skins – you don't need to be perfectionist about this, I normally remove about half. If the soup is too thick add a little water and bring it back up to temperature. Adjust the seasoning if necessary and then serve.

Vietnamese king prawns and sugar snaps

194 calories

Very quick and bursting with flavour!

Serves 2   Preparation time: 5 minutes   Cook time: 5 minutes

Quick & easy

200g (7oz) raw king prawns (king or jumbo shrimp) (152 cals)
salt and freshly ground black pepper
zest and juice of 1 lime (4 cals)
1 tsp fish sauce (4 cals)
½ tsp sugar (8 cals)
1 tsp olive oil (27 cals)
200g (7oz) sugar snaps (68 cals)
1 spring onion (scallion), trimmed and finely chopped (5 cals)
handful of fresh coriander (cilantro), chopped
20g (⅛ cup) salted peanuts, roughly chopped or bashed (120 cals)

- Dry the prawns (shrimp) with kitchen paper (paper towels) and season with salt and pepper.
- Put the zest of the lime into a small bowl and the juice of half the lime. Stir in the fish sauce and sugar.
- Heat the oil in a wide frying pan (skillet) over a high heat. When the oil is very hot, add the prawns, sugar snaps and spring onion (scallion) and stir-fry for 3 minutes. Reduce the heat and stir in the fish sauce mixture. Cook for 1 more minute or until the prawns are cooked through.
- Turn off the heat and toss through the coriander (cilantro) and peanuts. Serve immediately with the remaining lime juice drizzled over.

Roasted aubergine with spicy yogurt dressing

110 calories

Serves 2   Preparation time: 5 minutes   Cook time: 30 minutes

Vegetarian

1 medium aubergine (eggplant), about 300g/11oz, halved lengthways (45 cals)
1 tbsp olive oil (99 cals)
salt and freshly ground black pepper
3 tbsp low-fat plain yogurt (67 cals)
juice of ½ lemon (2 cals)
½ tsp paprika (3 cals)
1 garlic clove, peeled and crushed (3 cals)
small handful of fresh mint, chopped

- Preheat the oven to 220°C/200°C fan/425°F/Gas mark 7.
- Score a criss-cross pattern in the aubergine (eggplant) halves with the tip of a knife, the scores should be about 1cm (½in) deep.
- Sit the aubergines in a roasting tin (pan) and drizzle with the olive oil, then season generously with salt and pepper. Roast in the oven for 30 minutes, until tender.
- Meanwhile, make up the dressing by combining the yogurt, lemon juice, paprika and garlic in a small bowl.
- When you are ready to serve, place the aubergines on a plate, drizzle the dressing over and top with the mint.

Harissa spiced chickpeas on green beans

184 calories

Chickpeas make a nutty filling meal but they can be a little boring. Here is a deliciously simple way to serve them.

Serves 2   Preparation time: 3 minutes   Cook time: 7–9 minutes

Vegetarian, quick & easy

1 tbsp harissa paste (13 cals)
1 tbsp tomato purée (paste) (30 cals)
1 × 400g (14oz) can chickpeas, rinsed and drained (276 cals)
juice of ½ lemon (2 cals)
200g (7oz) fresh green beans, trimmed (48 cals)

- Heat the harissa and tomato purée (paste) in a frying pan (skillet) over a medium heat for 1–2 minutes, until it just starts to sizzle. Reduce the heat to low and stir in the chickpeas and lemon juice. Cook for 2–3 minutes, until warmed through.
- Cook the green beans in a pan of boiling water until just tender, about 4 minutes.
- Serve the chickpeas over the green beans.

Smoky BBQ chicken

197 calories

Don't be put off by the long list of ingredients, they are all storecupboard regulars. The quantities listed here are for two portions of sauce. It keeps in the fridge for at least a week (and is very addictive) so feel free to double up the portions and store in a covered pot.

Serves 2   Preparation time: 5 minutes   Cook time: 10–14 minutes

Quick & easy, barbecue or grill

1 tsp dark brown sugar (18 cals)
¼ tsp smoked paprika (2 cals)
½ tsp dried oregano (2 cals)
1 tsp cornflour (cornstarch) (18 cals)
1 tsp Dijon mustard (11 cals)
½ tsp maple syrup (13 cals)
¼ tsp Worcestershire sauce (1 cal)
1 tsp cider vinegar (1 cal)
½ tsp black treacle (blackstrap molasses) (10 cals)
pinch of salt
2 × 150g (5oz) skinless chicken breasts, scored lightly with a knife (318 cals)

- Preheat the grill (broiler) or barbecue to a medium–high setting.
- Simply mix together all the ingredients except the chicken in a small bowl. Add a little water if necessary to make it into a spreadable consistency.
- Spread the mixture over the chicken breasts, making sure you coat all sides.
- Grill (or barbecue) the chicken for 5–7 minutes on each side depending on thickness and check that the chicken is cooked through before serving.

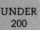

Chilled strawberries and Cointreau

99 calories

These succulent strawberries can be kept in the fridge for up to two days.

Serves 2   Preparation time: 5 minutes, plus chilling

250g (1¾ cups) strawberries, hulled and thickly sliced (68 cals)
1 tbsp Cointreau (48 cals)
zest of ½ orange (4 cals)
1 level tbsp caster (superfine) sugar (79 cals)

- Put the strawberries into a bowl with the Cointreau, orange zest and caster (superfine) sugar. Stir lightly to combine without breaking up the strawberries.
- Cover and refrigerate for about 1 hour for the flavours to develop. Spoon into dishes or goblets to serve.

Honey glazed pineapple

107 calories

Serves 4   Preparation time: 5 minutes   Cook time: 10 minutes

1 medium fresh pineapple (750g/1lb 10oz) (308 cals)
10g (2 tsp) butter (74 cals)
2 tsp runny honey (46 cals)
pinch of ground cinnamon

continued

- Remove the skin and core from the pineapple and cut the flesh into large chunks.
- Heat half the butter and 1 teaspoon of the honey in a wide frying pan (skillet). When they have melted together increase the heat, add the pineapple and fry for about 8 minutes, turning often, until caramelized.
- Reduce the heat to low and stir in the rest of the butter and honey and a pinch of cinnamon. When it is all melted together and sticky, serve immediately in a bowl or glasses.

Vanilla ice cream soda

109 calories

A very simple low-calorie treat, I used Green & Black's organic vanilla ice cream.

Serves 1 Preparation time: 2 minutes

300ml (1¼ cups) diet cream soda (3 cals)

1 heaped tablespoon (or scoop) (60g/2¼oz) best quality
vanilla ice cream (106 cals)

- Pour the cream soda into a large glass and top with the scoop of ice cream. Serve with a straw.

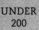
Raspberry sorbet

138 calories

This sorbet is so so simple.

Serves 4   Preparation time: 5 minutes, plus freezing

150g (scant ½ cup) redcurrant jelly (360 cals)
200g (1⅔ cups) raspberries (50 cals)
250g (generous 1 cup) 0% fat Greek yogurt (142 cals)

- Place all the ingredients in a food processor or blender and blend together until smooth.
- Transfer to a suitable container and freeze until firm. Remove from the freezer about 30 minutes before serving.

Peach Melba

141 calories

Serves 2   Preparation time: 10 minutes   Cook time: 5 minutes

Quick & easy

1 medium peach (36 cals)

2 heaped tablespoons (or scoops) (about 60g/2¼oz each) vanilla ice cream (212 cals)

100g (scant 1 cup) fresh raspberries (25 cals)

1 tsp icing (confectioners') sugar (10 cals)

- Half the peach and remove the stone (pit).
- Bring a small pan of water to the boil and poach the halved peach for about 5 minutes. A really ripe peach will take less time. Remove from the water and take off the skin.
- Place the raspberries in a sieve (strainer) and crush the raspberries through the sieve with the back of a fork. Stir in the icing (confectioners') sugar to the resulting raspberry syrup.
- Put scoops of ice cream on two serving plates, then balance the peaches on the top and pour on the raspberry sauce.

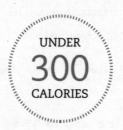

UNDER
300
CALORIES

Classic Greek salad

218 calories

Easy to knock up, this salad is great for a light fast day lunch or lunch box.

Serves 1 Preparation time: 5 minutes

Vegetarian, quick & easy

1 tsp extra virgin olive oil (27 cals)
1 tsp white wine vinegar (1 cal)
pinch of sugar (4 cals)
salt and freshly ground black pepper
2 fresh basil leaves, finely chopped
1 × 80g (3oz) bag mixed leaf salad (16 cals)
5cm (2in) piece cucumber, roughly diced (10 cals)
2 medium tomatoes, roughly diced (28 cals)
2 spring onions (scallions), trimmed and shredded (10 cals)
50g (1¾oz) light feta cheese, cut into small cubes (91 cals)
6 black olives, pitted (31 cals)

- In a small bowl, stir together the olive oil, vinegar, sugar, salt and pepper and basil leaves.
- Put the salad leaves in a wide bowl or container and lightly toss in the cucumber, tomatoes and spring onions (scallions). Drizzle over the dressing and toss again.
- Arrange the feta and black olives over the top and serve.

Tangy bulgur wheat and broad bean salad

295 calories

This is a great dish made using storecupboard and frozen ingredients. It's perfect for a lunch box.

Serves 1   Preparation time: 5 minutes   Cook time: 20 minutes

Vegetarian

50g (⅓ cup) cracked bulgur wheat (176 cals)
salt and freshly ground black pepper
50g (1¾oz) frozen broad (fava) beans (30 cals)
4 radishes, thinly sliced (4 cals)
¼ red onion, peeled and very thinly sliced (14 cals)
small handful of fresh mint, chopped (10 g) (4 cals)
zest and juice of 1 lime (4 cals)
½ small red chilli, deseeded and finely chopped (2 cals)
1 tsp extra virgin olive oil (27 cals)
1 tsp white wine vinegar (1 cal)
½ tsp English mustard (6 cal)
1 tsp runny honey (23 cals)

- Place the bulgur wheat in a bowl and season with salt and pepper. Pour on 100ml (scant ½ cup) just boiled water, then cover and leave to cook for 15 minutes until tender.
- Cook the broad (fava) beans in boiling water for 4–5 minutes, then combine the broad beans with the bulgur wheat and leave to cool.
- When the beans and bulgur wheat are cool, stir through the radishes, red onion and mint.
- In a small bowl, mix together the lime zest and juice, chilli, olive oil, vinegar, mustard and honey. Pour over the salad, then serve immediately or cover and keep refrigerated until needed.

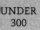
Italian courgette and tomato salad

263 calories

This is a simple and easy salad. Using thinly cut courgette (zucchini) gives the salad substance without the calories.

Serves 1   Preparation time: 10 minutes   Cook time: 5 minutes

Quick & easy

1 large or 2 small courgettes (zucchini) (250g/9oz), trimmed (45 cals)
20 cherry tomatoes, quartered (45 cals)
zest of ½ lemon (1 cal)
1 tbsp balsamic vinegar (12 cals)
1 tsp extra virgin olive oil (27 cals)
½ tsp olive oil (13 cals)
½ garlic clove, peeled and crushed (or ½ tsp garlic purée/paste) (2 cals)
salt and freshly ground black pepper
5 fresh basil leaves
½ ball light Italian mozzarella (75 g) (119 cals)

- Use a vegetable peeler or mandoline to cut your courgette (zucchini) into ribbons. Discard the first slice as it will be mainly skin. If using the vegetable peeler, make slices until you hit the seeds, then rotate and peel again.
- Mix the tomatoes, lemon zest, balsamic vinegar and extra virgin olive oil together in a bowl.
- In a wide frying pan (skillet), heat the olive oil over a medium–high heat. When hot, toss in the garlic and fry for 1 minute. Add the courgette, then season with salt and pepper and cook for 2 minutes. Give it a stir and cook for a further 1–2 minutes or until the courgette is cooked through yet firm.

continued

- Transfer the courgette to a serving bowl and pour the tomato mixture over. Tear the basil and mozzarella and arrange over the top. Serve immediately.

Avocado and bacon salad

274 calories

This is an oldie but a goodie!

Serves 1   Preparation time: 5 minutes   Cook time: 5 minutes

Quick & easy

15g (½oz) streaky bacon, chopped (about 1 slice) (50 cals)
¼ red onion, finely sliced (14 cals)
½ red (bell) pepper, finely sliced (26 cals)
1 × 80g (3oz) bag mixed leaf salad (16 cals)
½ ripe avocado, sliced (138 cals)
1 tsp extra virgin olive oil (27 cals)
juice of ¼ lemon (1 cal)
salt and freshly ground black pepper

- Heat a small frying pan (skillet) over a medium–high heat and fry the bacon until brown and crisp. Dry and cool on kitchen paper (paper towels).
- Using the oil left in the pan from the bacon, reduce the heat a little and fry the onion and red (bell) pepper for 5–7 minutes until tender and golden.
- Place the salad leaves in a wide bowl and mix through the onion and red pepper. Add the sliced avocado and drizzle with the olive oil and lemon juice. Season with salt and pepper and top with the crispy bacon.

Chicken salad with lemon pepper dressing

294 calories

Serves 1   Preparation time: 5 minutes   Quick & easy

1 tbsp low-fat crème fraîche (57 cals)
juice of ½ lemon (2 cals)
freshly ground black pepper
pinch of salt
pinch of sugar (4 cals)
1 x 80g (3oz) bag baby leaf or herb salad (16 cals)
5cm (2in) piece cucumber, finely sliced (10 cals)
1 medium tomato, sliced (14 cals)
1 cooked chicken breast (125g/4oz) (191 cals)

- Combine the crème fraîche, lemon juice, black pepper, salt and sugar in a small bowl.
- Arrange the salad leaves, cucumber and tomato in a wide bowl.
- Cut the chicken into thick slices and arrange on top of the salad. Drizzle the dressing over and serve.

Courgette 'pizza' bites

216 calories

This dish is such an easy guilt-free treat. If you don't have any garlic oil, crush about a quarter of a garlic clove and stir into the oil before using.

Serves 1   Preparation time: 5 minutes   Cook time: 5 minutes

Quick & easy

2 medium courgettes (zucchini) (54 cals)
2 tsp garlic oil (54 cals)
salt and freshly ground black pepper
2 medium tomatoes, finely chopped (28 cals)
50g (1¾oz) low-fat mozzarella, chopped (80 cals)
4 fresh basil leaves

- Preheat the grill (broiler) to a high setting.
- Cut the courgettes (zucchini) in half on the diagonal so you get 2 oval slices (about 1cm/½in thick) from each courgette.
- Put the garlic oil in a small bowl. Crumple up a piece of kitchen paper (paper towel), dip it into the oil and rub the courgette slices on both sides with the oil.
- Lay out the courgettes on a grill (broiler) pan and cook under the grill for 2 minutes on each side.
- Remove from the grill and distribute the chopped tomatoes over each slice of courgette.
- Next, top with the mozzarella and finally a basil leaf.
- Return to the grill and cook until the cheese starts to bubble.

Asparagus pile up

218 calories

Lots of good things – together at last!

Serves 1   Preparation time: 5 minutes   Cook time: 12 minutes

Quick & easy

1 large egg, pricked (91 cals)
100g (3½oz) fine asparagus (25 cals)
10 cherry tomatoes, quartered (22 cals)
1 tsp extra virgin olive oil (27 cals)
1 tsp balsamic vinegar (5 cals)
1 slice Parma ham (prosciutto), cut into pieces (27 cals)
5g (1 tsp) Parmesan cheese, finely grated (21 cals)
salt and freshly ground black pepper

- Bring a small saucepan of water to a fast boil. Slowly lower the egg into the water and cook for 7½ minutes. Remove the egg from the water and peel under cold running water. Set aside.
- Lightly cook the asparagus by plunging into boiling water and boiling for 4–5 minutes, until just tender.
- Mix together the cherry tomatoes with the olive oil and balsamic vinegar.
- Put the asparagus on a plate and pour the cherry tomatoes over. Next, add the Parma ham (prosciutto).
- Quarter the egg and add it to the pile. Finally, sprinkle on the Parmesan cheese and a generous seasoning of salt and pepper.

Courgette and feta fritters

260 calories

Serves 2   Preparation time: 15 minutes   Cook time: 8 minutes

Vegetarian, quick & easy

2 courgettes (zucchini), trimmed (54 cals)
3 spring onions (scallions), trimmed and finely chopped (15 cals)
100g (3½oz) light feta cheese, crumbled (182 cals)
little fresh parsley, chopped (5 g) (2 cals)
1 tsp dried mint (2 g) (6 cals)
½ tsp paprika (3 cals)
salt and freshly ground black pepper
1 level tbsp plain (all-purpose) flour (68 cals)
1 large egg, beaten (91 cals)
1 tbsp olive oil (99 cals)

- Coarsely grate the courgettes (zucchini) and lay out on kitchen paper (paper towels) to dry out. Leave for about 10 minutes, then pat the top of the courgette to get rid of any extra moisture.
- Mix the spring onions (scallions), crumbled feta, parsley, mint and paprika in a bowl. Season with salt and pepper and stir in the flour. Pour in the beaten egg and mix well. Finally, mix in the grated courgette.
- Heat the oil in a wide frying pan (skillet) over a medium-high heat. When hot, add 1 tablespoon scoops of the mixture to the pan, flattening each scoop with the back of the spoon as you go. The fritters need to be widely spaced so you may have to do this in 2 batches. Fry for about 2 minutes on each side until golden. Serve immediately.

Oven-baked sweet potato wedges with real aïoli

202 calories

I've discovered that it is far easier than I thought to make real mayonnaise. I use an electric mixer rather than a blender and it is somehow a lot easier and tidier.

Serves 2   Preparation time: 10 minutes   Cook time: 45 minutes

Vegetarian

2 small sweet potatoes (about 100g/3½oz each) (174 cals including skin)
salt and freshly ground black pepper
2 tsp sunflower oil (54 cals)
1 tbsp extra virgin olive oil (99 cals)
¼ garlic clove, peeled and crushed (1 cal)
1 large egg, separated, yolk only (73 cals)
juice of ½ lime (2 cals)

- Preheat the oven to 220°C/200°C fan/425°F/Gas mark 7.
- Peel and cut the sweet potatoes into large wedges. If you prefer you can leave the skin on the potatoes.
- Place the sweet potato wedges into a pan of cold, salted water and bring to the boil. Cook for 15 minutes from cold. Drain and leave to cool until they are cold enough to handle.
- Place the sweet potatoes in a roasting tray and pour on the oil. Toss through with your hands so that the potatoes are as covered as possible and season well. Bake in the oven for 25–30 minutes until crispy and golden.
- Meanwhile, prepare the aïoli. Mix the olive oil and garlic in a small dish or jug (pitcher).

continued

- Place the egg yolk in a clean bowl and, using an electric mixer, beat the egg yolk thoroughly. Add 2 drops of oil and mix again, then ever so slowly pour the oil into the yolk, beating constantly. Continue until you have an emulsion. Squeeze in the lime juice, still beating. The aïoli should have a colour and texture similar to custard. Scoop into two small dishes and set aside until needed.
- To serve, arrange the sweet potato wedges over two serving plates and put a bowl of aïoli on the side.

Super easy crushed chickpeas with Boursin

262 calories

Don't knock it until you've tried it! This incredibly easy crush takes just a few minutes to make and is very filling and flavoursome.

Serves 1   Preparation time: 2 minutes   Cook time: 3 minutes

Extra filling, quick & easy

1 tbsp (20g/¾oz) Boursin soft cheese (122 cals)
juice of ½ lime (2 cal)
1 tbsp water
½ × 400g (14oz) can chickpeas, rinsed and drained (138 cals)
salt and freshly ground black pepper

- Gently heat the Boursin, lime juice and water in a small frying pan (skillet). When the Boursin starts to melt tip in the chickpeas and heat for about 3 minutes, until the chickpeas are warmed through. Mash the chickpeas together with a masher or just a fork. You want them to be broken up and sticking together but not smooth. Season generously with salt and pepper. This can be served hot or cold.

Spicy bean burgers

202 calories per burger

These vegetarian burgers can be frozen before cooking. Simply freeze on a baking tray and then wrap in foil or store in an airtight container. Defrost before cooking.

Makes 4 burgers   Preparation time: 10 minutes, plus chilling
Cook time: 10 minutes

Freezer-friendly, vegetarian

1 × 400g (14oz) can cannellini beans, rinsed
and drained (259 cals)

2 tbsp (50g/1¾oz) red pesto (164 cals)

75g (½ cup) wholemeal (wholewheat) breadcrumbs (163 cals)

1 large egg (91 cals)

4 spring onions (scallions), trimmed and chopped (20 cals)

1 garlic clove, peeled and crushed (3 cals)

salt and freshly ground black pepper

4 tsp sunflower oil (1 tsp per burger) (108 calories)

- Use a potato masher to thoroughly mash the beans. Add the pesto, breadcrumbs, egg, spring onions (scallions) and crushed garlic. Add a little salt and pepper and mix well.
- Divide the mixture into 4 portions and form into balls. Place on a baking tray or plate. Squeeze the ball down with the palm of your hand to form a burger. For best results chill at this stage for about 30 minutes to help the burgers retain their shape.
- When you are ready to cook the burgers, heat the oil in a frying pan (skillet) over a medium heat. Add the burgers to the pan and cook for 4–5 minutes on each side until golden. Serve hot.

Caribbean casserole

251 calories

A flavoursome vegetarian casserole, this couldn't be simpler – you just
throw it all in!

Serves 4   Preparation time: 15 minutes   Cook time: 2½–6 hours

Vegetarian, freezer-friendly, slow cooking

1 large onion, peeled and chopped (86 cals)
1 red (bell) pepper, chopped (51 cals)
2 green chillies, deseeded and chopped (6 cals)
2 medium sweet potatoes, peeled and cut into wedges (150g/5oz) (261 cals)
1 × 400g (14oz) can chopped tomatoes (64 cals)
2 tbsp shop-bought salsa (12 cals)
1 × 200g (7oz) can pineapple chunks in juice, drained (137 cals)
1 cooking apple, peeled, cored and roughly chopped (35 cals)
250ml (generous 1 cup) vegetable stock (made with ½ cube) (18 cals)
1 × 400g (14oz) can butter (lima) beans, rinsed and drained (220 cals)
1 tbsp dark brown sugar (54 cals)
1 tbsp desiccated (dry unsweetened) coconut (60 cals)
1 tsp chilli powder
½ tsp ground cumin
½ tsp dried oregano (2 cals)
pinch of ground cinnamon

continued

- Preheat the oven to 160°C/140°C fan/325°F/Gas mark 3.
- Place all the ingredients in a large casserole dish, put on the lid and cook in the oven for 2½ hours. Check the water levels halfway through cooking. Alternatively, cook in a slow cooker for about 6 hours.

Lime and chilli prawns with salsa

229 calories

Serves 1   Preparation time: 10 minutes, plus standing

Quick & easy

1 medium tomato, diced (14 cals)
¼ red onion, peeled and finely diced (14 cals)
½ small red chilli, deseeded and finely chopped (2 cals)
1 tsp olive oil (27 cals)
juice of 1 lime (4 cals)
salt and freshly ground black pepper
150g (5oz) cooked prawns (shrimp), roughly chopped (148 cals)
handful of fresh coriander (cilantro), chopped
1 Little Gem (Boston) lettuce, separated into leaves (20 cals)

- Place the tomato, red onion and chilli in a small bowl and add the oil, lime juice and salt and pepper. Leave to mellow for 5 minutes.
- Combine the prawns (shrimp) and coriander (cilantro) in a bowl then mix in the marinated tomato and onion.
- Arrange the lettuce on a serving plate and scoop the prawns and salsa over.

Fiery coconut crab cakes

233 calories

These are very easy and delicious. I use canned crabmeat here for super simplicity.

Serves 1/makes 4–6 cakes   Preparation time: 5 minutes, plus chilling

Cook time: 2 minutes

Quick & easy

1 × 170g (6oz) can white crabmeat, drained (120g/4oz drained weight) (92 cals)
1 tbsp plain (all-purpose) flour (68 cals)
1 tbsp (10g/⅓oz) desiccated (dry unsweetened) coconut (60 cals)
2 slices jalapeño peppers (from a jar), chopped (4 cals)
pinch of sugar (4 cals)
juice of ½ lime (2 cals)
few sprays light oil (3 cals)
lime wedge, to serve

- Combine the crabmeat, flour, coconut, jalapeños, sugar and lime juice in a bowl, then form the mixture into 4–6 small balls. Place the balls on a baking tray and press down gently with the back of a fork to make a small patty. Cover with clingfilm (plastic wrap) and chill for 30 minutes until set.
- Heat a wide non-stick frying pan (skillet) over a high heat with a little spray oil. When hot, lift the patties into the pan, leaving as much space as you can between them and cook for about 1 minute on each side. They should be pleasingly golden and heated right through inside.
- Serve immediately with a wedge of lime on the side.

Seared scallops with garlicky potatoes

252 calories

This is fresh and easy.

Serves 2   Preparation time: 5 minutes   Cook time: 20 minutes

200g (7oz) new potatoes, halved (140 cals)

1 tbsp sunflower oil (99 cals)

1 garlic clove, peeled and crushed (3 cals)

freshly ground black pepper

¼ red onion, cut into half rings (14 cals)

50g (1¾oz) watercress (11 cals)

200g (7oz) fresh scallops, cut in half horizontally (236 cals)

juice of 1 lemon (4 cals)

- Boil the potatoes for about 12 minutes until just cooked through. Drain then leave to cool slightly on kitchen paper (paper towels) and blot dry.
- Heat the oil in a frying pan (skillet) over a medium heat and fry the potatoes, garlic and black pepper together until the potatoes are just browning. Remove the potato and garlicky goodness from the pan and place in a bowl with the red onion and watercress.
- Wipe the pan with kitchen paper to remove any excess oil and heat the pan over a high heat. When hot, add the scallops and fry for 1–2 minutes. They should be seared on both sides and just cooked through.
- Toss the cooked scallops into the potatoes and squeeze on the lemon juice before serving.

Olive chicken and broccoli

250 calories

Serves 2   Preparation time: 5 minutes   Cook time: 20 minutes

Quick & easy

2 × 150g (5oz) skinless chicken breasts (318 cals)
2 shallots (12 cals)
1 bay leaf
200g (7oz) head broccoli, cut into florets (66 cals)
1 tsp olive oil (27 cals)
1 garlic clove, peeled and finely sliced (3 cals)
1 small red chilli, deseeded and finely chopped (4 cals)
12 large black olives, pitted (62 cals)
2 tbsp light soy sauce (9 cals)

- Place the chicken breasts in the base of a lidded saucepan, together with 1 of the shallots cut in half and the bay leaf. Pour on boiling water until generously covered and bring to a gentle simmer for 5 minutes. Turn off the heat, put the lid on and leave the chicken to cook for a further 5 minutes. Check the chicken is cooked through before removing from the pan. Leave to cool slightly before cutting into slices.
- Boil the broccoli by submerging in boiling water and simmering for 6 minutes until tender. Drain and set aside.
- Chop the remaining shallot into fine half rings. Heat the olive oil in a wide frying pan (skillet) over a medium heat and lightly fry the shallot until golden and soft. Add the garlic and chilli and fry for a further 2 minutes.
- Stir in the cooked chicken and broccoli, together with the olives. Finally, add the soy sauce and warm through before serving.

Parmesan chicken

266 calories

Serves 2   Preparation time: 5 minutes   Cook time: 12 minutes

Quick & easy

20g (4 tbsp) Parmesan, finely grated (90 cals)
1 tsp plain (all-purpose) flour (17 cals)
salt and freshly ground black pepper
1 egg white (9 cals)
2 x 150g (5oz) skinless chicken breast, halved (318 cals)
70g (⅔ cup) peas, fresh or frozen (58 cals)
50g (1¾oz) baby spinach leaves (12 cals)
1 tsp extra virgin olive oil (27 cals)
1 tsp white wine vinegar (1 cal)

- Preheat the grill (broiler) to a medium setting.
- Loosely mix the Parmesan, flour and a little salt and pepper on a plate. Beat the egg white in a wide bowl.
- Dip each piece of chicken first in the egg white and then in the Parmesan, making sure it is lightly coated on both sides.
- Place the chicken pieces on a grill (broiler) tray and cook under the grill for 5–6 minutes on each side until golden and cooked through.
- While the chicken is cooking, cook the peas in boiling water for 6 minutes until tender.
- Drain the peas and return to the pan. Stir through the spinach, allowing it to wilt slightly in the heat. Add the olive oil and vinegar and stir through.
- Transfer to 2 serving plates and arrange 2 pieces of chicken each on top of the green vegetables.

Chicken 'burger' with Portobello bun

281 calories

Serves 1   Preparation time: 10 minutes   Cook time: 25 minutes

4 large Portobello mushrooms, about 75g (2½oz) each, washed (39 cals)
2 tsp olive oil (54 cals)
1 shallot, peeled and finely sliced (6 cals)
1 × 150g (5oz) skinless chicken breast, halved (159 cals)
½ garlic clove, peeled and finely chopped (2 cals)
1 medium tomato, chopped (14 cals)
2 jalapeño slices from a jar, chopped (2 cals)
1 tsp red wine vinegar (1 cal)
¼ Little Gem (Boston) lettuce, shredded (4 cals)

- Preheat the grill (broiler) to a medium setting.
- Cut the stalks off the mushrooms and chop the stalks finely.
- Heat half the oil in a small frying pan (skillet), add the shallot and slowly fry until tender, about 7 minutes.
- Rub the remaining oil over both sides of the chicken pieces and over the inside of the mushrooms.
- Place the mushrooms and chicken under the grill and cook for about 10–12 minutes, turning once, until the chicken is cooked through.
- Meanwhile, add the garlic, tomato, chopped mushroom stalks and jalapeños to the shallots and continue to fry for a further 5 minutes. Remove from the heat and stir through the vinegar.
- To make up your burgers, place 2 mushrooms face up on the serving plate. Add a little shredded lettuce and then put your grilled (broiled) chicken on top. Add a dollop of the mushroom salsa and place the other 2 mushrooms on the top. Serve immediately.

Lamb with quick Cumberland sauce

237 calories

This is a tasty and easy lamb dish, perfect for rustling up after work.

Serves 2   Preparation time: 5–8 minutes   Cook time: 10–15 minutes

Quick & easy

1 tsp olive oil (27 cals)
1 garlic clove, peeled and crushed (3 cals)
2 × 90g (3¼oz) lean lamb leg steaks (337 cals)
zest and juice of ½ orange (50 cals)
1 tbsp redcurrant jelly (20 g) (48 cals)
½ tsp English mustard (5 cals)
½ tsp Worcestershire sauce (2 cals)
1 tsp dark soy sauce (2 cals)

- Heat the oil in a frying pan (skillet) over a medium–high heat. When hot, add the garlic and fry for 1 minute before adding the lamb. Fry for 4–8 minutes on each side, depending on thickness and how you like your lamb.
- While the lamb is cooking, place the orange zest and juice, redcurrant jelly, mustard, Worcestershire sauce and soy sauce in a small bowl. Mush the redcurrant jelly with a fork and stir until combined.
- When the lamb is cooked, remove the pan from the heat. Add the sauce mixture to the lamb and turn the meat in the sauce until well coated.
- Rest the lamb in the sauce for about 2 minutes before serving.

Banana pancakes

251 calories

A simple treat for breakfast or any time of day!

Serves 1/makes 5 pancakes   Preparation time: 5 minutes
Cook time: 5 minutes

Quick & easy

1 large egg (18 cals for egg white)
1 medium banana, peeled (95 cals)
1 tbsp plain (all-purpose) flour (102 cals)
½ tsp vanilla extract (6 cals)
½ tsp baking powder (3 cals)
¼ tsp ground cinnamon
pinch of salt

- Separate the egg. We only need the egg white in this recipe.
- In a wide bowl, mash the banana thoroughly with a fork. Whisk in the egg white followed by the rest of the ingredients and combine until smooth.
- Heat a non-stick frying pan (skillet) over a medium-high heat. Once the pan is hot, spoon about 2 tablespoons of the mixture into the pan. Depending on the size of your pan, you may be able to cook 2–3 pancakes at the same time. Wait until each pancake starts to form bubbles on the surface, then flip. Depending on the size of your pancake it will take 1–2 minutes cooking on each side.
- Make all your pancakes in the same way and serve immediately.

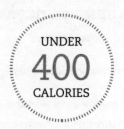

UNDER
400
CALORIES

Creamy salmon salad

309 calories

Serves 1   Preparation time: 5 minutes, plus standing   Cook time: 18 minutes

Quick & easy

1 skinless salmon fillet, about 130g (4½oz) (234 cals)

1 tsp very low-fat mayonnaise (14 cals)

1 tbsp low-fat plain yogurt (20 cals)

1 tbsp rice wine vinegar (3 cals)

2 fresh mint leaves, finely chopped

salt and freshly ground black pepper

1 × 80g (3oz) bag baby leaf or herb salad (16 cals)

2 radishes, thinly sliced (2 cals)

5cm (2in) piece cucumber, cut into chunks (10 cals)

2 spring onions (scallions), trimmed and sliced (10 cals)

- Preheat the oven to 200°C/180°C fan/400°F/Gas mark 6.
- Place the salmon fillet on a baking tray and bake in the oven for 16–18 minutes until just cooked through. Remove from the oven and set aside – the salmon is equally nice hot or cold in the salad.
- In a small bowl, mix the mayonnaise, yogurt, vinegar, mint and salt and pepper together and leave to stand for at least 5 minutes to allow the flavours to develop.
- Arrange the salad leaves on a serving plate and top with the radishes, cucumber and spring onions (scallions). Flake the salmon over the top and drizzle the dressing over.

Lamb tagine

303 calories

This delicious concoction is sweet and spicy. I have adapted the traditional recipe here to suit my own needs – it really works. Most of the ingredients are storecupboard favourites, so it is a breeze to put together.

Serves 4   Preparation time: 15 minutes   Cook time: 2–8 hours

Easy, freezer-friendly, slow cooking

1 tbsp vegetable oil (99 cals)
1 tbsp plain (all-purpose) flour, seasoned with salt and freshly ground black pepper (68 cals)
300g (11oz) extra lean diced lamb (459 cals)
1 medium onion, chopped (54 cals)
2 tsp mild chilli powder
1 tsp turmeric
1 tsp ground cumin
1 x 400g (14oz) can chopped tomatoes (64 cals)
500ml (generous 2 cups) lamb/chicken or vegetable stock (made with 1 cube) (35 cals)
100g (½ cup) pearl barley (360 cals)
1 tbsp shop-bought salsa (7 cals)
1 tbsp apricot jam (63 cals)
juice of 1 lime (4 cals)

- Preheat the oven to 180°C/160°C fan/350°F/Gas mark 4 if using. Heat the oil in a large lidded casserole dish over a high heat.
- Sprinkle the seasoned flour over the diced lamb and use your hands to mix it through and make sure all the surfaces of the meat are covered.

continued

- When the oil is hot, toss in the meat and fry for about 2 minutes without stirring. Then stir, turn and fry the other side for a further 2 minutes. Remove the lamb from the dish with a slotted spoon.
- Turn the heat down to low and add the onion. Stir in the spices, then add the chopped tomatoes and stock. Bring to the boil. Add the pearl barley and boil vigorously for 10 minutes.
- Return the lamb to the casserole. Stir in the salsa, jam and lime juice. Put the lid on and cook in the oven for 2 hours OR transfer to a slow cooker and cook on low for 6–8 hours.

Fragrant chicken

333 calories

This is a delicate and quick dish.

Serves 2   Preparation time: 10 minutes   Cook time: 25 minutes

Quick & easy

1 tsp olive oil (27 cals)
1 small onion, peeled and finely chopped (22 cals)
½ tsp cumin seeds
½ tsp turmeric
300ml (1¼ cups) fresh chicken stock (21 cals)
½ lemon (2 cals)
2 × 150g (5oz) skinless chicken breasts, diced (318 cals)
200g (7oz) new potatoes, quartered (140 cals)
few strands of saffron
10g (2 tsp) butter (74 cals)
12 large black olives, pitted (62 cals)
4 fresh basil leaves, roughly chopped
salt and freshly ground black pepper

- Heat the oil in a pan over a low heat, add the onion and sweat for 7–8 minutes. Add the cumin seeds and turmeric and fry for 1–2 minutes until aromatic.
- Pour in the chicken stock and bring to a gentle simmer. Add the lemon zest then cut out the flesh of the lemon, roughly chop and add to the pan.
- Add the chicken, potatoes and saffron. Bring back to simmering point and cook gently for 10 minutes until the potatoes are tender and the chicken is cooked through. Remove the chicken and potatoes from the pan and keep warm.
- Increase the heat under the pan to high and stir in the butter, olives, basil and salt and pepper. Bubble over a high heat for 2–4 minutes until the sauce is a little thicker and glossy. Pour the sauce over the chicken and potatoes and serve immediately.

Rainy day stew

312 calories

As its name suggests this recipe is a light and easy stew for a warm but wet summer's evening.

Serves 2   Preparation time: 5 minutes   Cook time: 40 minutes

Easy, freezer-friendly

1 litre (4 cups) chicken stock (fresh is best here) (70 cals)

1 leek, trimmed and sliced (26 cals)

2 Cumberland sausages, sliced into 2cm (¾in) pieces (207 cals)

1 red chilli, deseeded if preferred and sliced (4 cals)

1 Parmesan rind (for flavour only, removed after cooking)

2 bay leaves

continued

½ tsp dried mixed herbs or small handful of fresh basil
and/or parsley if available

1 courgette (zucchini), halved and sliced (27 cals)

50g (scant ½ cup) peas, fresh or frozen (42 cals)

50g (1¾oz) macaroni (or other small pasta) (174 cals)

2 medium tomatoes, diced (29 cals)

salt and freshly ground black pepper

10g (2 tbsp) fresh Parmesan, grated (45 cals)

- Heat the chicken stock in a large saucepan with the leek, sausages, chilli, Parmesan rind, bay leaves and dried herbs. Bring to a gentle simmer and cook for about 25 minutes.
- Add the courgette (zucchini), peas and macaroni and simmer for a further 10–15 minutes until the pasta and peas are tender.
- Remove the Parmesan rind and bay leaves from the pan and add the tomatoes and any fresh herbs if using.
- Serve in large bowls and season generously. Sprinkle the grated Parmesan over the top.

AUTUMN

AUTUMN RECIPES

Under 200 calories

Cheesy herb muffins

Spanish scrambled eggs

Apple and celeriac soup

Creamy mushroom and white wine soup

Carrot and coriander soup

Yellow pepper soup

Garlicky mushrooms

Oven-baked celeriac chips

Cheesy swiss chard bake

Roasted pumpkin with goat's cheese

Quick home-made beans with chorizo

Pork steaks with mushrooms

Cinnamon apples

Apple and blackberry compote

Lemon kisses

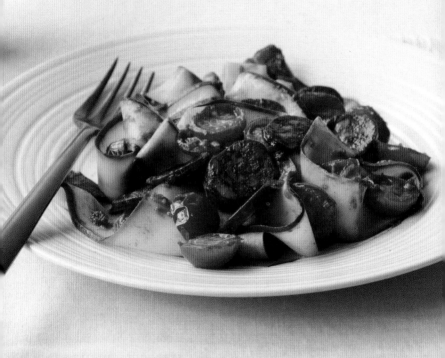

Courgette ribbons with tomato and chorizo sauce: 158 calories (p50).

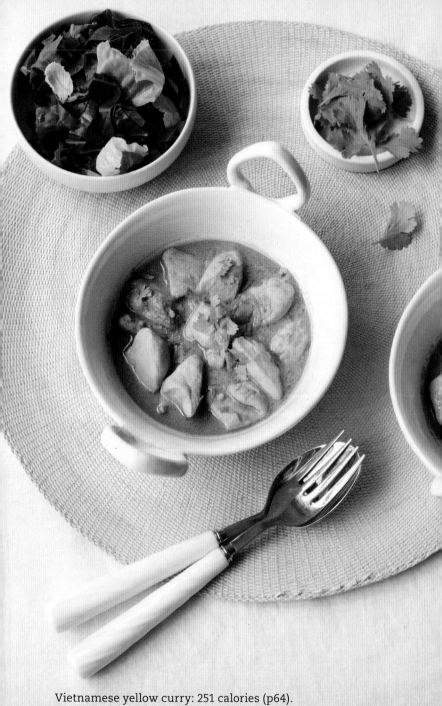

Vietnamese yellow curry: 251 calories (p64).

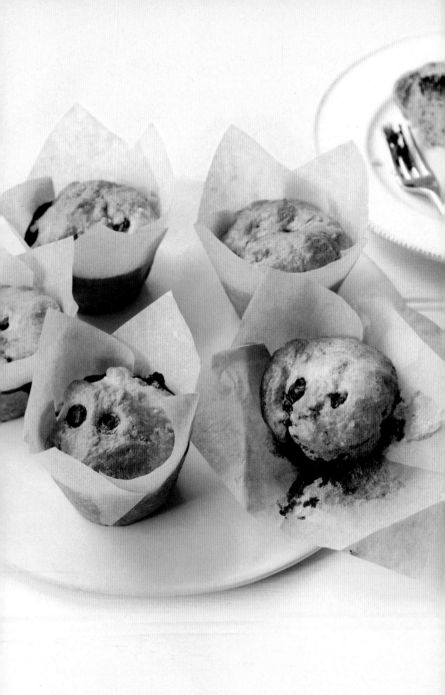

Healthy blueberry bran muffins: 139 calories (p87).

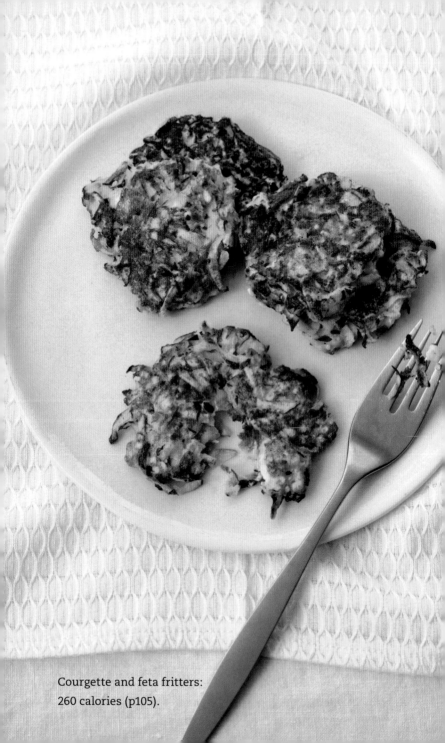

Courgette and feta fritters:
260 calories (p105).

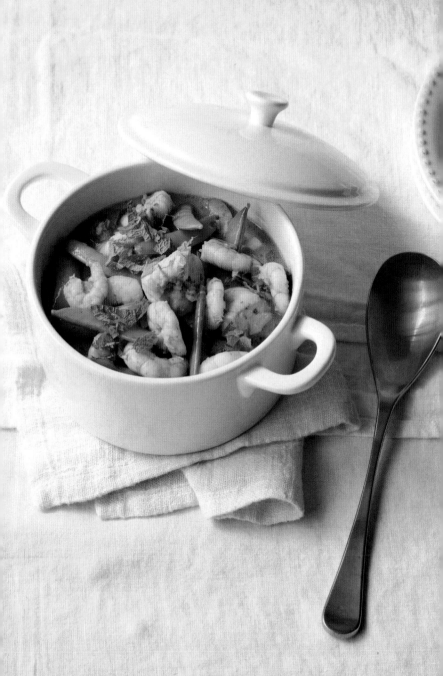

Monkfish and prawn stew: 281 calories (p149).

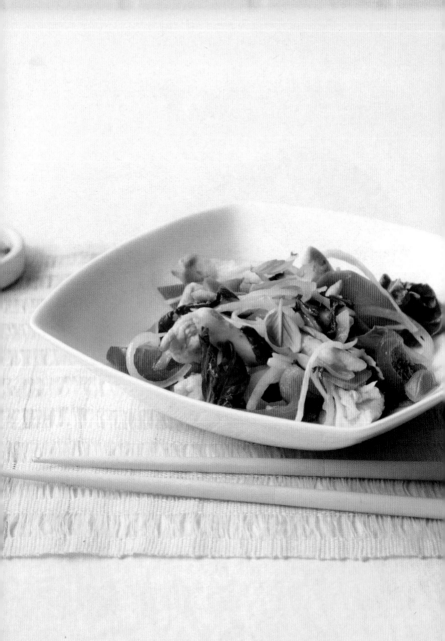

Chinese chicken stir-fry: 306 calories (p165).

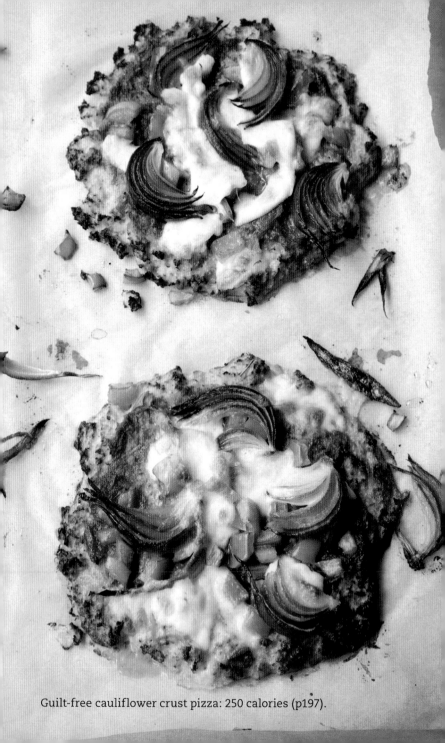

Guilt-free cauliflower crust pizza: 250 calories (p197).

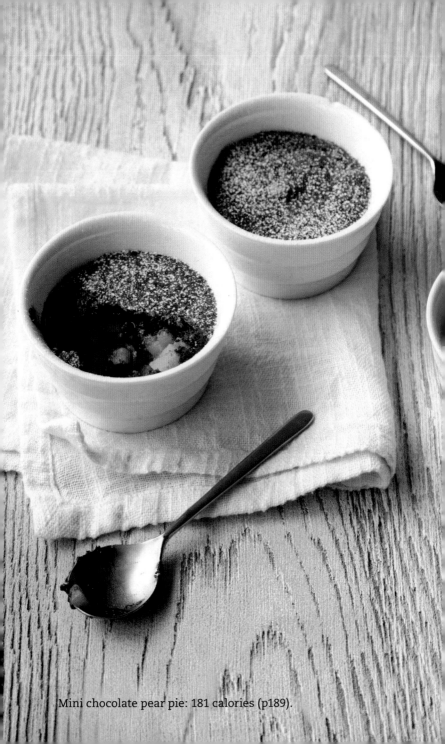

Mini chocolate pear pie: 181 calories (p189).

Under 300 calories

So simple pasta soup
Anchovy and egg salad
Smoked mackerel and lentil salad
Monkfish and prawn stew
Thai baked salmon
Slow-cooked chicken casserole
Honey lemon chicken with broccoli
Chicken with baked spaghetti squash
Pork with pears and walnuts
Seared beef with blackberry sauce
Mushroom stroganoff
Lebanese chickpea curry
Apple and ginger crunch
Gooseberry cobbler

Under 400 calories

Steamed salmon with spicy kale
Chicken poached in white wine
One pot lemon chicken
Chinese chicken stir-fry
Ginger chicken with lentils
Italian beef courgette lasagne
Autumn vegetable crumble

BACK TO SCHOOL.
BACK TO DIET.

The back-to-school season and often the back-to-diet season too after letting your guard down over the summer.

Don't despair, Autumn is the season of mushrooms and squashes: both extremely low calorie and filling. I have included plenty of imaginative recipes for these ingredients. Pork steaks with mushrooms (see page 142) is a particular favourite with my other half as it is simply not 'diety' at all. Meals made with squash or pumpkin also have the advantage of being similar to potatoes but with only about half the calories. If you can get hold of spaghetti squash you can make amazing pasta dishes – without the pasta. And if you can't resist a comforting lasagne, my lasagne recipe, made with sliced courgette in place of the pasta sheets, does not compromise on flavour one bit.

As it is harvest season, there are loads of fruit and vegetables around. Small portions of fruit such as apples and blackberries make a tasty and not very high calorie treat. A small apple has 53 calories and a healthy handful (50g/⅓ cup) of blackberries has only 24 calories. I like to freeze blackberries when I go picking (or buy them in frozen packets from the supermarket) and eat them like sweets straight from the freezer!

Autumn is the time to explore the rich variety of fruit and vegetables open to you. Vegetables in particular are so low in calories that you can knock up some amazing large plates of food that will satisfy the biggest of appetites. It is also the time to start stocking the freezer. Make a big pot of Apple and celeriac soup (see page 133) and freeze it in individual portions. You will be so grateful to your autumn planning when you can't move your fingers for the cold in January.

Menu plans for diet days

Use these planners to inspire your cooking on diet days. It's amazing how much good food you can eat for under 500–600 calories.

Just work out whether you want three small meals/breakfast and dinner/lunch and dinner on your diet days and choose the right planner for you. If you need more help working out which plan is right for you have a look at *What kind of dieter are you?* (see page 6).

Feel free to swap a recipe for another with a similar calorie content if necessary.

MENU PLANS FOR DIET DAYS: WOMEN (AUTUMN)

WOMEN: 3 SMALL MEALS

	Breakfast	Lunch	Dinner	Cals
Day 1	Cheesy herb muffin (page 131) 131 cals	Apple and celeriac soup (page 133) 62 cals	Chinese chicken stir-fry (page 165) 306 cals	499
Day 2	Apple and blackberry compote (page 144) 60 cals	Quick home-made beans with chorizo (page 141) 180 cals	Thai baked salmon (page 150) (239) 100g (3½oz) green beans (24) 263 cals	503

WOMEN: BREAKFAST AND DINNER

	Breakfast	Dinner	Cals
Day 1	Spanish scrambled eggs (page 132) 192 cals	Pork steak with mushrooms (page 142) (198) 100g (3½oz) broccoli (33) Apple and blackberry compote (page 144) (60) 291 cals	483
Day 2	Cinnamon apples (page 143) 139 cals	Slow-cooked chicken casserole (page 151) (220) 200g (7oz) new potatoes (140) 360 cals	499

	Lunch	Dinner	Cals
	WOMEN: LUNCH AND DINNER		
	Lunch	**Dinner**	**Cals**
Day 1	Carrot and coriander soup (page 135) *116 cals*	Seared beef with blackberry sauce (page 156) (248) Small baked sweet potato (130) *378 cals*	**494**
Day 2	Garlicky mushrooms (page 137) *99 cals*	Pork with pears and walnuts (page 155) (281) 150g (5oz) new potatoes (3 small) (105) *386 cals*	**485**

MENU PLANS FOR DIET DAYS: MEN (AUTUMN)

	Breakfast	Lunch	Dinner	Cals
	MEN: 3 SMALL MEALS			
	Breakfast	**Lunch**	**Dinner**	**Cals**
Day 1	Spanish scrambled eggs (page 132) *192 cals*	Garlicky mushrooms (page 137) *99 cals*	Pork with pears and walnuts (page 155) (281) 100g (3½oz) mangetout (snow peas) (32) *313 cals*	**604**
Day 2	Omelette made with 2 large eggs and ½ tsp olive oil *192 cals*	Carrot and coriander soup (page 135) *116 cals*	Smoked mackerel and lentil salad (page 148) *290 cals*	**598**

MEN: BREAKFAST AND DINNER

	Breakfast	Dinner	Cals
Day 1	2 large boiled eggs (178) Slice of wholemeal (wholewheat) toast (110) 288 *cals*	Chinese chicken stir-fry (page 165) 306 *cals*	594
Day 2	Spanish scrambled eggs (page 132) 192 *cals*	Thai baked salmon (page 150) (239) 200g (7oz) new potatoes (4 small) (140) 100g (3½oz) green beans (24) 403 *cals*	595

MEN: LUNCH AND DINNER

	Lunch	Dinner	Cals
Day 1	So simple pasta soup (page 146) 293 *cals*	Chicken poached in white wine (page 163) 322 *cals*	615
Day 2	Mushroom stroganoff (page 157) 207 *cals*	Seared beef with blackberry sauce (page 156) (248) 200g (7oz) new potatoes (4 small) (140) 388 *cals*	595

AUTUMN RECIPES

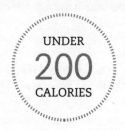

UNDER
200
CALORIES

Cheesy herb muffins

131 calories per muffin

These muffins are great for breakfast or as a light snack.

Makes 12   Preparation time: 10 minutes   Cook time: 25 minutes

180ml (scant 1 cup) skimmed (skim) milk (58 cals)

juice of ½ lemon (2 cals)

80g (3oz) frozen spinach (4 cubes) (18 cals)

100g (¾ cup) plain (all-purpose) flour (341 cals)

100g (⅔ cup) wholemeal self-raising (wholewheat
self-rising) flour (310 cals)

small handful of chives, finely chopped (10 g) (2 cals)

small handful of fresh parsley, finely chopped (10 g) (3 cals)

40g (⅓ cup) Parmesan cheese, finely grated (181 cals)

½ tsp bicarbonate of soda (baking soda)

2 tsp baking powder (14 cals)

pinch of salt

1 large egg (91 cals)

75g (⅓ cup) butter, melted (558 cals)

continued

- Pre-heat the oven to 200°C/180°C fan/400°F/Gas mark 6. Line a 12-hole muffin tin (pan) with paper cases.
- Combine the milk and lemon juice in a bowl or jug (pitcher) and leave to rest for 5 minutes.
- Reheat the spinach in the microwave for about 1 minute, then squeeze out any water.
- Mix the flours, herbs, cheese, bicarbonate of soda (baking soda), baking powder and salt together in a large bowl, then stir in the spinach.
- In another bowl, whisk the egg and melted butter together, then add the curdled milk.
- Pour the liquid ingredients over the dry ingredients and stir together. Do not overmix, it should stay rather lumpy.
- Spoon a fat teaspoon of batter into each paper case and bake in the oven for 20–25 minutes until just browning on top. Remove from the oven and leave to cool in the tin.
- These are equally good hot or cold.

Spanish scrambled eggs

192 calories

Serves 1   Preparation time: 10 minutes   Cook time: 15 minutes

Vegetarian

1 tsp olive oil (27 cals)
1 shallot, peeled and finely diced (6 cals)
1 garlic clove, peeled and sliced (3 cals)
½ green (bell) pepper, deseeded and diced (24 cals)
½ tsp dried mixed herbs
pinch of salt
pinch of sugar (4 cals)
2 medium tomatoes, chopped (28 cals)
1 large egg (91 cals)
1 egg white (9 cals)

continued

- Heat the oil in a frying pan (skillet) over a low heat. Add the shallot, garlic, pepper, herbs, salt and sugar and stir-fry for about 8 minutes until soft and golden. Add the chopped tomatoes, then turn up the heat to medium and bubble for a further 5 minutes.
- Meanwhile, whisk the egg and egg white together. Pour the eggs into the frying pan and stir constantly until they thicken like scrambled eggs. Serve immediately.

Apple and celeriac soup

62 calories

Easy, tasty and exceptionally low in calories.

Serves 4   Preparation time: 10 minutes   Cook time: 25–30 minutes

Vegetarian, freezer-friendly

1 onion, peeled and chopped (54 cals)
1 large cooking apple, peeled and chopped (54 cals)
½ medium celeriac, about 350g (12oz), peeled and chopped (63 cals)
1 litre (4 cups) vegetable stock (fresh or made with 2 cubes) (70 cals)
1 tsp curry powder (7 cals)
1 tsp mixed herbs
freshly ground black pepper

- Put the onion, apple and celeriac in a large saucepan and pour over the stock. Bring to the boil. Add the curry powder and mixed herbs then reduce the heat and simmer for 20–25 minutes until tender.
- Blend until smooth, then return the soup to the pan and bring back to temperature before serving. Generously season with pepper before serving.

Creamy mushroom and white wine soup

106 calories

Serves 4   Preparation time: 10 minutes   Cook time: 30 minutes

Vegetarian

1 tsp olive oil (27 cals)
1 large onion, peeled and finely chopped (86 cals)
1 garlic clove, peeled and finely sliced (3 cals)
400g (14oz) mushrooms, sliced (52 cals)
600ml (2½ cups) vegetable stock (fresh or made with 1 cube) (35 cals)
1 bay leaf
10g (2 tsp) butter (74 cals)
200ml (generous ¾ cup) white wine (66 cals)
50g (3 tbsp/¼ cup) light soft cheese (78 cals)
handful of fresh parsley (10g/⅓oz), chopped (3 cals)
salt and freshly ground black pepper

- Heat the oil in a large saucepan, add the onion and gently fry for 7 minutes. Add the garlic and fry for a further 2 minutes.
- Add about three-quarters of the mushrooms, turn in the oil then add the stock and bay leaf. Put a lid on and simmer for 15 minutes until the mushrooms are soft.
- Remove the bay leaf and blend until smooth.
- Heat the butter in a frying pan (skillet). When the butter has melted, toss in the remaining mushrooms and fry, turning once, until lightly browned.
- Return the blended soup to the pan and stir in the wine, cheese and parsley. Reheat gently and season to taste. Serve the soup with the fried mushrooms scattered on the top.

Carrot and coriander soup

116 calories

This classic soup is a breeze to make.

Serves 4   Preparation time: 10 minutes   Cook time: 25 minutes

Freezer-friendly, vegetarian

1 large onion, peeled and chopped (86 cals)
500g (1lb 2oz) carrots, about 6 medium (175 cals)
1 small potato (100g/3½oz), peeled and chopped (75 cals)
1 tsp ground coriander
1 litre (4 cups) vegetable stock (fresh or made with 2 cubes) (70 cals)
large handful of fresh coriander (cilantro) (15g/½oz) (3 cals)

To serve

freshly ground black pepper
2 tsp extra virgin olive oil (54 cals)

- Simply place the onion, carrots, potato and ground coriander in a large saucepan and pour in the stock. Bring to the boil, reduce the heat and simmer for 20 minutes until tender.
- Blitz in a blender or food processor with the fresh coriander until smooth. Return the soup to the pan and reheat gently.
- Serve with lashings of black pepper and a drizzle (½ teaspoon) of extra virgin olive oil.

Yellow pepper soup

157 calories

Serves 4   Preparation time: 20 minutes   Cook time: 50–60 minutes

Vegetarian, freezer-friendly

4 large yellow (bell) peppers, deseeded and halved (177 cals)
1 tbsp olive oil (99 cals)
10g (2 tsp) butter (74 cals)
1 onion, peeled and finely chopped (54 cals)
1 garlic clove, peeled and finely chopped (3 cals)
1 red chilli, deseeded and finely chopped (2 cals)
1 large/2 small potatoes (200g), peeled (150 cals)
1 tsp dried mixed herbs
1 litre (4 cups) vegetable stock (fresh or made with 2 cubes) (70 cals)
freshly ground black pepper

- Preheat the oven to 220°C/200°C fan/425°F/Gas mark 7.
- Place the yellow (bell) peppers skin side up on a baking tray and drizzle with the olive oil. Bake in the oven for 10–15 minutes until soft and blackened.
- Transfer the peppers to a bowl and cover with clingfilm (plastic wrap). Allow to steam in their own heat for 10 minutes, then peel off the skin and roughly chop.
- Meanwhile, heat the butter in a large saucepan over a low heat until melted. Toss in the onion, garlic and chilli and fry gently for 10 minutes. Add the (bell) peppers and any remaining juices from the baking tray or bowl.
- Add the potatoes, dried herbs and stock and bring to the boil. Reduce the heat and simmer for 30–45 minutes.
- Blitz in a blender or food processor until smooth, then return to the pan and reheat gently. Season generously with black pepper before serving.

Garlicky mushrooms

99 calories

This is a low-calorie quickie for when the hunger calls.

Serves 1   Preparation time: 5 minutes   Cook time: 7 minutes

Vegetarian, quick & easy

1 tsp olive oil (27 cals)

5g (1 tsp) butter (37 cals)

250g (9oz) mushrooms, sliced (32 cals)

1 garlic clove, peeled and crushed (3 cals)

handful of fresh parsley (10g/⅓oz), chopped (3 cals)

- Heat the oil and butter together slowly in a pan until the butter has melted. Turn the heat to high, add the mushrooms and fry for about 3 minutes until golden all over. Reduce the heat to low, add the garlic and stir-fry for 2 more minutes. Remove from the heat and stir in the parsley.

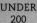
Oven-baked celeriac chips

112 calories

Serves 2   Preparation time: 10 minutes, plus drying   Cook time: 32 minutes

Vegetarian

1 medium celeriac (700g/1½lb) (126 cals)
1 tbsp sunflower oil (99 cals)
1 tsp cumin seeds
salt and freshly ground black pepper

- Preheat the oven to 220°C/200°C fan/425°F/Gas mark 7.
- Cut off the top and bottom of the celeriac. Use a sharp knife to cut off the tough knobbly skin. Cut the celeriac in half lengthways, before cutting into thick slices. Cut the slices again to get large chips.
- Bring a large pan of salted water to the boil and toss in the celeriac. Boil for 2 minutes then drain. Leave to dry a little in the colander before tipping back into the empty pan. Add the oil, cumin seeds and salt and pepper. Toss thoroughly using your hands.
- Pour the chips onto a baking tray and cook in the oven for 30 minutes, turning once.

Cheesy Swiss chard bake

184 calories

Serves 4   Preparation time: 15 minutes   Cook time: 40 minutes

Vegetarian

500g (1lb 2oz) Swiss or rainbow chard (95 cals)
freshly ground black pepper
400ml (1¾ cups) skimmed (skim) milk (128 cals)
20g (1½ tbsp) butter (149 cals)
1 tbsp plain (all-purpose) flour (68 cals)
2 tsp Dijon mustard (22 cals)
30g (scant ¼ cup) light feta cheese, crumbled (50 cals)
1 tbsp light soft cheese (55 cals)
30g (¼ cup) Cheddar, grated (124 cals)
10g (2 tbsp) Parmesan, finely grated (45 cals)

- Preheat the oven to 200°C/180°C fan/400°F/Gas mark 6.
- Cut the stalks off the chard leaves and chop into chunks. Place in a microwaveable bowl with 1 tablespoon water. Cover with clingfilm (plastic wrap) and microwave for 1 minute, then rest for 1 more minute.
- Arrange in a layer on the base of a large shallow baking dish.
- Chop the chard leaves roughly and arrange over the stalks. Grind over some black pepper.
- Pour the cold milk into a non-stick saucepan and add the butter and flour. Turn the heat to high and use a plastic balloon whisk to whisk the sauce from cold until the sauce thickens and bubbles. Remove from the heat and keep whisking for 1 more minute.
- Stir in the mustard, feta, soft cheese, half the Cheddar and half the Parmesan. Leave for a few minutes for the cheeses to melt into the sauce.
- Pour over the chard, pushing it to the edges with the back of a spoon if necessary and top with the remaining Cheddar and Parmesan.
- Bake in the oven for 30 minutes until golden.

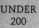

UNDER 200

Roasted pumpkin with goat's cheese

172 calories

Serves 2   Preparation time: 10 minutes   Cook time: 25 minutes

Vegetarian

1 garlic clove, whole (2 cals)
450g (1lb) pumpkin, peeled, deseeded and cut into chunks (58 cals)
1 tbsp olive oil (99 cals)
salt and freshly ground black pepper
100g (3½oz) baby spinach (25 cals)
50g (¼ cup) soft goat's cheese, chopped into cubes (160 cals)

- Preheat the oven to 210°C/190°C fan/400°F/Gas mark 6½.
- Leave the garlic in its skin and crush with the flat side of a knife.
- Place the garlic in a large bowl with the pumpkin and olive oil. Toss the oil through the pumpkin using a metal spoon or your hands.
- Transfer the pumpkin mixture to a roasting tray and season with salt and pepper. Roast in the oven for 20–25 minutes, turning once, until tender and browned.
- Remove the tray from the oven. Squeeze out the garlic with the back of a fork and discard the skin. Toss the spinach through. Transfer to serving dishes and arrange the goat's cheese over the top. Season generously with black pepper and serve immediately.

Quick home-made beans with chorizo

180 calories

Easy and warming, this is even better than the real thing!

Serves 2   Preparation time: 10 minutes   Cook time: 20 minutes

Extra filling, quick & easy

1 x 400g (14oz) can haricot beans, rinsed and
drained (258 cals)

250ml (generous 1 cup) chicken or veg stock
(fresh or made with ½ cube) (17 cals)

1 tsp tomato purée (paste) (8 cals)

1 tsp tomato ketchup (8 cals)

½ tsp Worcestershire sauce (2 cals)

½ tsp sugar (8 cals)

1 tsp red wine vinegar (1 cal)

20g (¾oz) chorizo, thinly sliced (58 cals)

- Put all the ingredients except the chorizo in a small saucepan and bring to the boil. Reduce the heat to low and cook gently for 10 minutes.
- While the beans are cooking, fry the chorizo in a frying pan (skillet) over a medium heat for 2–3 minutes until browned. You won't need to add any oil as the chorizo will release its own as it starts to cook.
- Add the chorizo and any fat from the pan to the beans and simmer for a further 5 minutes.
- The beans can be served immediately but keep well in the fridge for up to two days.

Pork steaks with mushrooms

198 calories

This dish might just get you in the mood for Christmas – it's made from tangerines and cranberry jelly.

Serves 2   Preparation time: 5 minutes   Cook time: 20 minutes

Quick & easy

2 tsp sunflower oil (54 cals)
2 × 100g (3½oz) lean pork steaks (240 cals)
100g (3½oz) mushrooms, sliced (13 cals)
1 heaped tsp paprika (14 cals)
1 tbsp cranberry jelly (24 cals)
juice of 2 tangerines (13 cals)
1 tsp red wine vinegar (1 cal)
1 tsp (5g) butter (37 cals)

- Heat the oil in a large frying pan (skillet) over a medium-high heat. When hot, add the pork steaks and fry for 2 minutes on each side. At this stage the pork should be browned but not cooked through.
- Remove the pork from the pan and fry the mushrooms for about 5 minutes until soft.
- Return the pork to the pan and add the paprika, cranberry jelly, tangerine juice and vinegar. Bring to a gentle simmer and stir to dissolve the cranberry jelly. Simmer for 5 minutes, turning the pork halfway through, until the meat is cooked.
- Remove the pork and mushrooms from the pan. Turn the heat up to medium and stir in the butter. Bubble for 2 minutes until the sauce is glossy.

Cinnamon apples

139 calories

A quick to cook autumnal treat.

Serves 1   Preparation time: 2 minutes   Cook time: 3 minutes

Quick & easy

10g (2 tsp) butter (74 cals)
½ tsp ground cinnamon
1 eating apple, cored and sliced (52 cals)
1 tsp (5g) maple syrup (13 cals)

- Melt the butter in a frying pan (skillet) over a low heat. Stir in the cinnamon.
- Turn the heat up to medium and add the apples. Sizzle for 1–2 minutes on each side until just beginning to brown.
- Serve piled on a plate with the maple syrup drizzled over the top.

Apple and blackberry compote

60 calories

Serves 4   Preparation time: 10 minutes   Cook time: 20 minutes

Freezer-friendly

2 large cooking apples (108 cals)	
juice of 1 lemon (4 cals)	
1 tbsp caster (superfine) sugar (79 cals)	
200g (1⅓ cups) blackberries (50 cals)	

- Peel, core and slice the apples. As the apples are prepared, put them into a large non-stick saucepan with a squeeze of lemon juice. This will limit the discoloration of the apples.
- Add 2 tablespoons water to the apples along with the caster (superfine) sugar. Bring the apples to the boil then reduce the heat to medium. Put the lid on and cook for 15 minutes, stirring every 5 minutes to stop them sticking.
- Stir in the blackberries and cook for a further 5–10 minutes. The blackberries should be tender but just holding their shape.
- Spoon into 4 separate ramekins. This dish can be served hot or cold.

Lemon kisses

80 calories per biscuit (cookie)

These cute little macaroon biscuits (cookies) are a teeny tiny treat. Store in an airtight container in the fridge for two days or in the freezer. I can eat these from frozen if the need takes me!

Makes 20 biscuits   Preparation time: 15 minutes, plus drying

Cook time: 15 minutes

Freezer-friendly

| 200g (1¾ cups) icing (confectioners') sugar (786 cals) |
| 100g (generous 1 cup) ground almonds (612 cals) |
| 3 large eggs (egg whites only) (49 cals) |
| pinch of salt |
| 40g (scant ¼ cup) caster (superfine) sugar (158 cals) |
| few drops yellow food colouring |
| zest of 1 lemon (1 cal) |

- Whizz the icing (confectioners') sugar and ground almonds in a food processor until you have a fine dust.
- Using an electric whisk, beat the egg whites with the salt until it forms stiff peaks. Add the caster (superfine) sugar slowly, beating all the time, until stiff and glossy. Whisk in the food colouring and lemon zest.
- With a metal spoon, fold the icing sugar and almonds into the egg whites. Do this slowly and gently until well-combined. Line two baking sheets with greaseproof paper or silicone sheets.
- Spoon teaspoons of the mixture onto the lined baking trays, leaving as much space as you can between them. Leave the mixture to dry for about 30 minutes – you should be able to touch the surface without leaving a fingerprint.
- Preheat the oven to 170°C/150°C fan/325°F/Gas mark 3.
- Bake in the oven for 12–14 minutes. Leave to cool completely on the tray before storing in an airtight container.

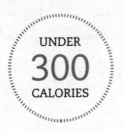

UNDER
300
CALORIES

So simple pasta soup

293 calories

Filled fresh pasta has slightly less calories than normal pasta and is used here sparingly.

Serves 4   Preparation time: 10 minutes   Cook time: 25 minutes

Vegetarian, quick & easy

1 tsp olive oil (27 cals)

1 large onion, peeled and finely chopped (86 cals)

2 garlic cloves, peeled and finely chopped (6 cals)

2 medium carrots, peeled and finely chopped (70 cals)

1 litre (4 cups) vegetable stock (fresh or made with
2 stock cubes) (70 cals)

1 x 400g (14oz) can chopped tomatoes (64 cals)

100g (scant 1 cup) frozen peas (66 cals)

100g (3½oz) asparagus, trimmed and chopped into
big pieces (25 cals)

300g (11oz) sundried tomato and mozzarella tortelloni
(760 cals)

continued

- Heat the olive oil in a large saucepan, add the onion, garlic and carrots and fry for 5 minutes until starting to soften. Add the stock and chopped tomatoes and bring to the boil. Reduce the heat and simmer for 10 minutes before adding the peas. Simmer for a further 5 minutes.
- Add the asparagus and simmer for 2 minutes. Finally, add the pasta and simmer for a further 3 minutes. Serve immediately.

Anchovy and egg salad

245 calories

Serves 2   Preparation time: 10 minutes   Cook time: 30 minutes

1 red (bell) pepper (54 cals)
1 green (bell) pepper (26 cals)
2 large eggs, pricked (182 cals)
1 garlic clove, peeled and crushed (3 cals)
1 tbsp olive oil (99 cals)
1 tbsp red wine vinegar (2 cals)
pinch of sugar (4 cals)
salt and freshly ground black pepper
6 anchovy fillets (60g/2¼oz), drained (115 cals)
1 tbsp capers (2 cals)
handful of fresh parsley (10g/⅓oz), roughly chopped (3 cals)

- Preheat the oven to 200°C/180°C fan/400°F/Gas mark 6.
- Place the red and green (bell) peppers on a baking sheet and roast in the oven for 20 minutes.
- Bring a saucepan of water to a fast boil. Gently lower the eggs into the water and cook for 7½ minutes for soft-boiled or 10 minutes for hard-boiled. Remove the eggs from the water and peel under cold running water. Set aside.

continued

- To make the dressing, mix together the crushed garlic, olive oil, vinegar and sugar. Season generously with salt and pepper.
- When the peppers are cooked, leave until just cool enough to handle, then remove as much skin as you can, but don't worry if you need to leave a bit on the pepper. Cut out the head and seeds and discard. Cut into strips and arrange on a serving plate.
- Quarter the eggs and add to the plate. Add the anchovies and sprinkle over the capers and parsley. Finally dress the salad with the garlic dressing and serve while still warm.

Smoked mackerel and lentil salad

290 calories

Serves 2   Preparation time: 5 minutes

Quick & easy

1 x 80g (3oz) bag mixed salad leaves (16 cals)
20 cherry tomatoes, halved (45 cals)
100g (½ cup) ready-to-eat Puy lentils (137 cals)
juice of ½ lemon, plus an extra squeeze (2 cals)
1 tsp extra virgin olive oil (27 cals)
salt and freshly ground black pepper
100g (3½oz) smoked mackerel fillets (354 cals)

- Place the salad leaves in a serving bowl and add the cherry tomatoes and lentils.
- Mix the lemon juice, olive oil and salt and pepper in a small bowl. Pour over the salad and toss lightly. Flake the mackerel over the top and squeeze over a little extra lemon juice before serving.

Monkfish and prawn stew
281 calories

Monkfish is a meaty fish that does not break up on cooking.

Serves 4   Preparation time: 15 minutes   Cook time: 1 hour 15 minutes

1 tsp sunflower oil (27 cals)

500g (1lb 2oz) skinless, boneless monkfish fillet,
cut into chunks (330 cals)

juice of 1 lime (4 cals)

2 red chillies, deseeded (4 cals)

4 garlic cloves, peeled (12 cals)

5cm (2in) piece of fresh ginger, peeled and
roughly chopped (9 cals)

1 tsp ground coriander

large bunch of fresh coriander (cilantro) (15g/½oz) (3 cals)

1 tbsp sesame oil (99 cals)

1 x 400ml (14fl oz) can light coconut milk (292 cals)

500ml (generous 2 cups) fish or vegetable stock
(fresh or made from 1 cube) (35 cals)

250g (9oz) raw king prawns (king or jumbo shrimp),
peeled and deveined (190 cals)

150g (5oz) sugar snaps (51 cals)

2 pak choi, roughly chopped (57 cals)

1 tbsp fish sauce (12 cals)

few fresh mint leaves, chopped (optional)

few basil leaves, chopped (optional)

- Heat the sunflower oil in a large saucepan or casserole dish and brown the monkfish on both sides. You may need to do this in 2 batches but it won't take longer than 1 minute on each side. Remove the monkfish to a plate and squeeze over the lime juice.

continued

- Use a food processor or hand blender to chop the chillies, garlic, ginger and coriander. Blend to a rough paste with the sesame oil.
- Heat the saucepan or casserole over a medium heat and stir-fry the chilli paste for 1 minute. Pour in the coconut milk and stock and bring to the boil. Return the monkfish to the pan. Cook on the lowest setting on the hob or in the oven at 170°C/150°C fan/325°F/ Gas mark 3 for 1 hour.
- Return the stew to a low simmer on the hob. Add the prawns (shrimp), sugar snaps, pak choi and fish sauce. Simmer for 10 minutes. Stir through the fresh herbs before serving.

Thai baked salmon

239 calories

Salmon is so simple to bake in the oven. If you top this with some simple Thai herbs and spices you can have an unusual and healthy dish. Note that I suggest you use pre-prepared purées for some of the Thai ingredients here – it makes it even simpler.

Serves 2   Preparation time: 5 minutes   Cook time: 18–20 minutes

Quick & easy

handful of fresh coriander (cilantro) (10g/⅓oz), chopped (3 cals)
zest and juice of ½ lime (3 cals)
½ lemongrass stalk, shredded or 1 tsp lemongrass purée (paste) (2 cals)
1cm (½in) piece of fresh ginger, peeled and grated or 1 tsp ginger purée (paste) (5 cals)
½ tsp mild chilli powder
pinch of salt
2 skinless salmon fillets, about 130g (4½oz) each (468 cals)

continued

- Preheat the oven to 200°C/180°C fan/400°F/Gas mark 6.
- In a small bowl, mix together all the ingredients except the salmon.
- Place the salmon fillets on a baking tray and rub the herb and spice mixture all over the top and sides of the salmon.
- Bake in the oven for 18–20 minutes until the salmon is just cooked through.

Slow-cooked chicken casserole

220 calories

This is a great recipe for just throwing everything in a pan and leaving it alone for a few hours. It's equally good on the hob, in the oven or in a slow cooker.

Serves 4   Preparation time: 10 minutes   Cook time: 2–8 hours

Easy, freezer-friendly, slow cooking

1 onion, peeled and chopped (54 cals)

2 carrots, peeled and roughly chopped (70 cals)

4 celery sticks, trimmed and sliced (20 cals)

2 garlic cloves, peeled and sliced (6 cals)

1 small swede (rutabaga) (180g/6½oz), peeled and roughly chopped (43 cals)

4 skinless, boneless chicken thighs, about 360g (12¾oz) (392 cals)

2 tbsp tomato purée (paste) (60 cals)

200ml (generous ¾ cup) red wine (136 cals)

1 × 400g (14oz) can tomatoes (64 cals)

400ml (1¾ cups) chicken stock (fresh or made with 1 stock cube) (35 cals)

2 bay leaves

salt and freshly ground black pepper   *continued*

- Put the onion, carrots, celery, garlic and swede (rutabaga) in the base of a large casserole dish or slow cooker dish. Place the chicken thighs in a layer over the vegetables, then spread the tomato purée (paste) over the chicken. Pour in the red wine, canned tomatoes and chicken stock, then tuck the bay leaves into the sauce and season well with salt and pepper.

On the hob
- Cook on the smallest ring and the lowest setting for 2–2½ hours, with the lid on, stirring every hour or so. Remove the lid if the sauce is too thin or add a little water if it looks a little dry.

In the oven
- Preheat the oven to 140°C/120°C fan/275°F/Gas mark 1 and cook for about 4 hours. Check an hour before the end of the cooking time and either remove the lid if it looks a little wet or add some water if it looks dry.

In the slow cooker
- Cook in the slow cooker on low for 6–8 hours.

- Stir well and adjust the seasoning if necessary before serving.

Honey lemon chicken with broccoli

276 calories

Serves 1   Preparation time: 5 minutes   Cook time: 10 minutes

Quick & easy

juice of ½ lemon (2 cals)
1 tsp balsamic vinegar (5 cals)
1 tsp extra virgin olive oil (27 cals)
1 tsp runny honey (23 cals)
salt and freshly ground black pepper
1 tsp olive oil (27 cals)

continued

1 × 150g (5oz) skinless chicken breast, cut in half (159 cals)

½ head broccoli, about 100g (3½oz), cut into florets (33 cals)

- Begin by preparing your serving dish. It should be wide with a lip and able to hold the chicken and broccoli comfortably. Put the lemon juice, vinegar, extra virgin olive oil, honey and salt and pepper in the dish and whisk together with a fork. Set aside.
- Heat the olive oil in a frying pan (skillet) over a medium–high heat. When hot, add the chicken pieces and fry for 6–8 minutes until golden and cooked through. As soon as it is cooked, transfer to the serving dish and toss in the dressing.
- Meanwhile, bring a pan of water to the boil and plunge in the broccoli. Cook for 6 minutes until tender. Drain and combine with the chicken and dressing.
- Leave the dish for 2 minutes before serving to allow the flavours to combine.

Chicken with baked spaghetti squash

256 calories

If you can't find any spaghetti squash, try making this with any other type of squash. Cut the squash into large cubes and roast in the oven for 30 minutes, then prepare the dish in the same way.

Serves 4   Preparation time: 30 minutes   Cook time: 30 minutes

1 medium spaghetti squash, about 500g/1lb 2oz,
halved lengthways and deseeded (115 cals)

1 tbsp olive oil (99 cals)

1 onion, peeled and finely chopped (54 cals)

2 garlic cloves, peeled and crushed (6 cals)

1 carrot, peeled and finely chopped (35 cals)

2 celery sticks, trimmed and finely chopped (10 cals)

continued

| 400g (14oz) diced chicken breast (424 cals) |
| 2 medium tomatoes, roughly chopped (28 cals) |
| 1 egg (76 cals) |
| 1 tsp English mustard (11 cals) |
| salt and freshly ground black pepper |
| 40g (⅓ cup) Parmesan, grated (166 cals) |

- Preheat the oven to 220°C/200°C fan/425°F/Gas mark 7.
- Bake the spaghetti squash face down on a baking tray in the oven for 30 minutes or until skin is soft and the threads of squash come out easily with a fork. Leave to cool.
- Meanwhile, heat the olive oil in a wide pan, add the onion, garlic, carrot and celery and fry for 5–10 minutes until soft. Turn up the heat to medium and add the chicken. Fry for 4–6 minutes until cooked, turning once. Toss in the tomatoes and cook for a further 2 minutes. Remove the pan from the heat.
- Use a fork to separate the squash from its skin and add the threads to the cooked chicken.
- In a small bowl, whisk together the egg, mustard, salt and pepper and about two-thirds of the Parmesan.
- Fill a large bowl with very hot water for 1–2 minutes until warm.
- When you are ready to serve the dish, pour out the water from the bowl and pour in the egg mixture. Immediately add the chicken, vegetables and squash and toss thoroughly, preferably using clean hands. This method of tossing beaten egg through the cooked chicken and squash gently coddles the egg but does not cook it fully. If you would prefer your egg to be completely cooked through, add the beaten egg mixture to the pan together with the squash, stir thoroughly and cook for 1–2 minutes.
- Serve immediately with a little extra Parmesan and freshly ground black pepper sprinkled over.

Pork with pears and walnuts

281 calories

Serves 2   Preparation time: 3–5 minutes   Cook time: 15 minutes

Quick & easy

20g (¼ cup) walnuts, roughly chopped (138 cals)
1 tsp sunflower oil (27 cals)
2 shallots, peeled and cut into eighths (12 cals)
2 pears, quartered and cored (120 cals)
1 tsp runny honey (23 cals)
1 fresh rosemary sprig (or ½ tsp dried) (2 cals)
2 × 100g (3½oz) lean pork steaks (240 cals)

- Heat a wide frying pan (skillet) over a high heat. Toss in the walnuts and toast for about 2 minutes, shaking once or twice to make sure they are evenly toasted. Remove to a plate and set aside.
- Add the oil and shallots to the pan and reduce the heat to medium. Fry the shallots for 3 minutes before adding the pears, honey and rosemary. Cook for another 3–5 minutes until starting to caramelise.
- Push the shallots and pears to the side and add the pork steaks. Fry for 5–8 minutes, turning once until browned and cooked to your liking. Serve with the toasted walnuts sprinkled over.

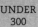
Seared beef with blackberry sauce

248 calories

The blackberries add a certain zing to this simple dish.

Serves 2   Preparation time: 5 minutes   Cook time: 15 minutes

Quick & easy

1 tsp olive oil (27 cals)
2 × 150g (5oz) lean beef escalopes (scallops) (375 cals)
salt and freshly ground black pepper
2 tsp balsamic vinegar (10 cals)
100ml (scant ½ cup) beef stock (fresh preferably or made with ¼ cube) (9 cals)
1 tbsp redcurrant jelly (48 cals)
1 tbsp port (12 cals)
1 garlic clove, peeled and crushed (3 cals)
50g (⅓ cup) blackberries, fresh or frozen (12 cals)

- Heat the oil in a frying pan (skillet) over a medium–high heat. Season the beef with the salt and pepper and add to the hot oil. Cook the beef for 4–8 minutes each side. The cooking time will depend on the thickness of the meat and how rare you like it. Remove the meat from the pan and set aside.
- Turn the heat down a little and add the vinegar, stock, redcurrant jelly, port and garlic. Bubble and stir for a few minutes to allow the sauce to reduce a little. Stir in the blackberries and cook for several minutes until tender. Return the meat to the pan and warm through before serving.

Mushroom stroganoff

207 calories

This is a great simple mid-week supper for one.

Serves 1   Preparation time: 10 minutes, plus steeping
Cook time: 15 minutes

Vegetarian, quick & easy

3 (1g) dried porcini mushrooms (3 cals)
3 sprays light oil (3 cals)
½ small red onion, peeled and finely chopped (11 cals)
1 garlic clove, peeled and finely chopped (3 cals)
1 tsp cornflour (cornstarch) (18 cals)
250g (9oz) mushrooms, sliced (32 cals)
2 fresh thyme sprigs
½ tsp paprika (3 cals)
1 tsp Dijon mustard (11 cals)
100ml (scant ½ cup) white wine (66 cals)
1 tbsp low-fat crème fraîche (57 cals)
salt and freshly ground black pepper

- First, put the porcini mushrooms in a small cup or bowl and just cover with boiling water. Leave to steep for at least 15 minutes.
- In a wide frying pan (skillet), heat the spray oil and lightly fry the onion and garlic for 3–5 minutes until softened.
- Turn the heat to low and add 1 tablespoon water. Sprinkle the cornflour (cornstarch) on top and cook gently while stirring continuously for 1 minute. Add the mushrooms, thyme, paprika and mustard and stir. Gradually stir in the wine and bring to a gentle simmer.
- Finely chop the softened porcini mushrooms and add to the pan, then cook for 10 minutes. Stir in the crème fraîche and season to taste. Serve immediately.

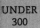

Lebanese chickpea curry

262 calories

This dish is unusual and very filling.

Serves 2   Preparation time: 10 minutes   Cook time: 40 minutes

Vegetarian, extra filling, freezer-friendly

1 tsp olive oil (27 cals)
1 onion, peeled and chopped (54 cals)
1 garlic clove, peeled and finely chopped (3 cals)
2 tsp ground cumin
¼ tsp ground cinnamon
2 tsp ground coriander
1 tbsp tomato purée (paste) (30 cals)
1 tsp harissa paste (4 cals)
½ red (bell) pepper, deseeded and diced (27 cals)
1 x 200g (7oz) can chickpeas (or half 400g/14oz can), rinsed and drained (138 cals)
40g (scant ¼ cup) red lentils (dry weight), rinsed (127 cals)
1 potato (170g/6oz), peeled and diced (75 cals)
500ml (generous 2 cups) vegetable stock (fresh or made with 1 cube) (35 cals)
juice of 1 lemon (3 cals)

- Heat the oil in a large saucepan, add the onion and fry for 7–8 minutes until translucent. Add the garlic and fry for 1 more minute. Stir in the spices, tomato purée (paste) and harissa paste, then add the diced pepper and fry for 3 minutes.
- Add the chickpeas, lentils, potato, stock and lemon juice. Bring to the boil, reduce the heat slightly and simmer vigorously for 10 minutes, before reducing the heat and simmering gently for a further 15 minutes.

Apple and ginger crunch

275 calories

Serves 6   Preparation time: 15 minutes   Cook time: 30 minutes

3 large cooking apples (161 cals)
juice of 1 lemon (4 cals)
1 tbsp caster (superfine) sugar (79 cals)
2 tbsp crystallized (candied) ginger, chopped (138 cals)
75g (scant 1 cup) porridge (rolled) oats (267 cals)
1 tbsp ground almonds (92 cals)
1 tbsp pine nuts (103 cals)
4 tbsp runny honey (276 cals)
2 tbsp demerara (raw brown) sugar (158 cals)
50g (4 tbsp) butter (372 cals)

- Preheat the oven to 200°C/180°C fan/400°F/Gas mark 6.
- Peel and core the apples and cut into thin slices. Arrange the apple slices over the base of a baking dish, squeezing on a little lemon each time you add more apples to help prevent discoloration.
- Sprinkle on the sugar and crystallized (candied) ginger and stir in lightly.
- Put the oats, almonds, pine nuts, honey and demerara (raw brown) sugar in a bowl. Melt the butter in the microwave or small saucepan and pour over the oat mixture. Mix well then spoon over the apples and ginger. Bake in the oven for 30–40 minutes.

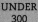
Gooseberry cobbler

242 calories

Serves 6   Preparation time: 25 minutes   Cook time: 40 minutes

800g (1¾lb) gooseberries, washed, topped and tailed (trimmed) (152 cals)
100g (½ cup) caster (superfine) sugar (394 cals)
2 tbsp elderflower cordial (87 cals)
140g (1 cup) plain (all-purpose) flour (477 cals)
2 tsp baking powder (13 cals)
1 tbsp demerara (raw brown) sugar (79 cals)
30g (2 tbsp) butter, cut into cubes and kept in fridge until needed (223 cals)
100ml (scant ½ cup) low-fat plain yogurt (56 cals)

- Preheat the oven to 190°C/170°C fan/375°F/Gas mark 5.
- Place the gooseberries, caster (superfine) sugar and elderflower cordial in a baking dish. Cover with foil and bake in the oven for 15 minutes.
- Meanwhile, prepare the cobbler topping. Place the flour, baking powder and demerara (raw brown) sugar in a large bowl and stir together.
- Add the cold butter and rub in with your fingers until it resembles fine breadcrumbs.
- Mix the yogurt and 50ml (scant ¼ cup) water together in a small bowl or jug (pitcher).
- Pour the thinned yogurt over the dry mix and loosely combine.
- Spoon tablespoons of the mixture over the fruit but do not smooth over and bake in the oven for 25–30 minutes.

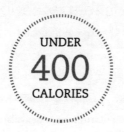

UNDER
400
CALORIES

Steamed salmon with spicy kale

327 calories

Don't be put off by the number of spices in this dish. If you don't have one or two just leave them out. If you are really pressed, try cooking the kale with 2 teaspoons of medium curry powder instead of all the spices.

Serves 2   Preparation time: 10 minutes   Cook time: 15 minutes

For the salmon:

½ tsp cumin seeds

few black peppercorns

bay leaf

2 skinless salmon fillets, about 130g (4½oz) each (468 cals)

For the kale:

1 tsp sunflower oil (27 cals)

½ tsp cumin seeds

½ tsp mustard seeds

1 tsp desiccated (dry unsweetened) coconut (18 cals)

½ tsp chilli powder

¼ tsp ground ginger (3 cals)

continued

½ tsp turmeric
½ tsp ground coriander
pinch of salt
200g (7oz) kale, shredded (66 cals)
100g (scant 1 cup) frozen peas (66 cals)
generous handful of fresh coriander (cilantro) (15g/½oz), roughly chopped (4 cals)
juice of ½ lemon (2 cals)

- In a small saucepan, heat the cumin seeds until they start to sizzle and toast. Remove from the heat. Add the peppercorns and bay leaf to the pan then lay the salmon on the top. Add just enough water to the pan to cover the salmon and bring the water to the boil. When boiling, reduce the heat and cook for 5–6 minutes until the salmon is cooked through. Remove the salmon from the pan and set aside.
- For the kale, heat the oil in a large lidded frying pan (skillet) over a medium–high heat. Add the cumin seeds, mustard seeds and coconut and fry for 1 minute until sizzling nicely.
- Stir in the rest of the spices and then the kale. Add the peas along with 2 tablespoons water. Put the lid on the pan and cook slowly for 6 minutes until the kale and peas are just cooked.
- Flake the salmon into large chunks into the pan. Add the fresh coriander (cilantro) and lemon juice, then warm through for 1–2 minutes before serving.

Chicken poached in white wine

322 calories

Yes! This is as good as it sounds.

Serves 1   Preparation time: 5 minutes   Cook time: 15 minutes

Quick & easy

1 tsp olive oil (27 cals)

½ garlic clove, peeled and crushed (2 cals)

2 spring onions (scallions), trimmed and sliced (10 cals)

½ tsp dried mixed herbs

1 x 150g (5oz) skinless chicken breast, halved (159 cals)

100ml (scant ½ cup) dry white wine (66 cals)

1 tbsp light soft cheese (25 cals)

small handful of fresh parsley (10g/⅓oz), chopped (3 cals)

- Heat the oil, garlic, spring onions (scallions) and dried mixed herbs in a small lidded frying pan (skillet) or saucepan for 1–2 minutes until sizzling. Add the chicken and cook for about 4 minutes until the first side turns golden.
- Turn the chicken over and add the white wine. Put the lid on and turn the heat to low. Let the chicken continue to cook in the wine for a further 5 minutes. Check that the chicken is cooked through before removing from the pan and covering.
- Bring the remaining liquid in the pan back up to simmering and stir in the soft cheese. Bubble for 2–3 minutes until you get a pleasingly thick sauce. Stir in the parsley and pour over the chicken.

One pot lemon chicken

395 calories

This dish has a very appetizing lemon colour.

Serves 4   Preparation time: 5 minutes   Cook time: 25 minutes

Quick & easy

1 lemon
1 tsp olive oil (27 cals)
4 × 150g (5oz) skinless chicken breasts (636 cals)
1 red onion, peeled and cut into wedges (54 cals)
2 tsp medium curry powder (14 cals)
1 tsp turmeric
200g (1 cup) basmati rice (718 cals)
500ml (generous 2 cups) hot chicken stock (made with 1 cube) (35 cals)
200g (7oz) cauliflower, cut into small florets (68 cals)
200g (7oz) green beans, fresh or frozen, trimmed (48 cals)
1 handful of fresh coriander (cilantro) (10g/⅓oz), chopped (optional) (3 cals)

- Wash the lemon in hot soapy water and dry. Cut in half lengthways and then cut into very thin slices.
- Using a large lidded frying pan (skillet) or casserole dish, heat the oil over a medium–high heat. When hot, add the chicken and red onion and brown the chicken on all sides.
- Stir in the curry powder, turmeric and rice, then pour in the hot stock.
- Add the cauliflower, beans and sliced lemon to the pan. Bring to the boil, reduce the heat and simmer with the lid on for 10 minutes. The chicken should be cooked through and the rice tender. Stir in the coriander (cilantro) and serve.

Chinese chicken stir-fry

306 calories

The slightly strange marinade for the chicken really works and gives the dish a Chinese takeaway feel.

Serves 2   Preparation time: 15 minutes, plus marinating
Cook time: 20 minutes

1 small egg white (7 cals)

2 tsp cornflour (cornstarch) (36 cals)

2 × 150g (5oz) skinless chicken breasts, cut into strips (318 cals)

1 tsp Thai fish sauce (nam pla) (4 cals)

juice of 1 lime (4 cals)

1 tsp vegetable oil (27 cals)

½ red (bell) pepper, deseeded and cut into large chunks (27 cals)

2.5cm (1in) piece of fresh ginger, peeled and grated (20 cals)

1 shallot, peeled and thinly sliced (6 cals)

1 garlic clove, peeled and thinly sliced (3 cals)

1 red chilli, deseeded and sliced (2 cals)

300g (11oz) bag mixed vegetable stir-fry (158 cals)

8 fresh basil leaves

- Whisk together the egg white and 1 teaspoon of cornflour (cornstarch) with a fork. Tip in the chicken and stir to coat. Leave to marinate for 15 minutes.
- Remove the chicken from the marinade and pat dry with kitchen paper (paper towels).
- Combine the fish sauce, lime juice, 2 tablespoons water and the rest of the cornflour.

continued

- Heat the oil in a wok or wide heavy-based frying pan (skillet) over a medium–high heat. When hot, toss in the chicken and stir-fry for 4–6 minutes until just cooked. Remove the chicken from the pan.
- Turn the heat to maximum and stir-fry the (bell) pepper, ginger, shallot, garlic and chilli for 2 minutes. Add the bagged veg and stir-fry for another 2 minutes until tender. Pour in the fish sauce mix and add the chicken and basil leaves. Heat through and serve immediately.

Ginger chicken with lentils

370 calories

Serves 2   Preparation time: 5 minutes   Cook time: 10 minutes

Extra filling, quick & easy

2 × 150g (5oz) skinless chicken fillets, cut into chunks (318 cals)
salt and freshly ground black pepper
1 tsp sunflower oil (27 cals)
10g (2 tsp) butter (74 cals)
1 large thumb of fresh ginger, peeled and finely grated (20 g) (10 cals)
1 garlic clove, peeled and crushed or finely grated (3 cals)
1 carrot, peeled and coarsely grated (35 cals)
200g (1 cup) ready-to-eat Puy lentils (274 cals)

- Season the chicken with salt and pepper.
- Heat the sunflower oil and butter together in a wide frying pan (skillet) over a medium–high heat. When hot, toss in the chicken and fry for 4–6 minutes, turning once, until just cooked.
- Turn the heat to high, stir in the ginger and garlic and fry for 1 more minute before turning the heat to low. Stir in the carrot and cook for a minute before adding the lentils. Cook slowly for a further few minutes until the lentils have warmed through.

Italian beef courgette lasagne

303 calories

This delicious lasagne is made using thinly sliced courgette in place of the lasagne sheets. As always with lasagne there are quite a few steps but it is all worth it. This lasagne freezes well so can be stored in individual pieces and reheated in the microwave.

Serves 6   Preparation time: 30 minutes, plus standing

Cook time: 1¾ hours

Freezer-friendly

1 tsp olive oil (27 cals)
1 onion, peeled and finely chopped (54 cals)
500g (1lb 2oz) extra-lean minced (ground) beef (870 cals)
1 garlic clove, peeled and finely chopped (3 cals)
1 × 400g (14oz) can chopped tomatoes (64 cals)
1 tbsp tomato ketchup (29 cals)
1 tsp dried mixed herbs
6 courgettes (zucchini) (162 cals)
salt
400ml (1¾ cups) skimmed (skim) milk (128 cals)
20g (1½ tbsp) butter (149 cals)
1 tbsp plain (all-purpose) flour (68 cals)
1 tbsp light soft cheese (55 cals)
30g (¼ cup) Cheddar, grated (124 cals)
20g (4 tbsp) Parmesan, finely grated (83 cals)

continued

- First make your Bolognese sauce in a large saucepan or casserole dish. Heat the oil over a low–medium heat and fry the onion for 5 minutes. Turn up the heat a little and add the beef and garlic. Fry, stirring constantly until all the meat has browned. Add the chopped tomatoes, ketchup and dried herbs and simmer, with the lid off, for 30–45 minutes.

- Next prepare the courgettes (zucchini). Slice the courgettes very thinly, discarding the first and last slice of skin. Each slice should be 2–4 mm (⅛in) thick. A mandoline or the right attachment on your food processor would make this job easier.

- Lay the first few slices of courgette out on kitchen paper (paper towels) and sprinkle with a little salt. Place another sheet of kitchen paper on top and add more courgette and salt. Repeat, making a small tower of courgette, until it has all been salted. Leave for 10–30 minutes.

- Rinse in a colander and blot dry with more kitchen paper.

- To make the cheese sauce, place the skimmed milk in a non-stick saucepan. Add the butter and flour. Turn the heat to high and whisk, using a plastic balloon whisk, constantly until thickened. Remove from the heat and stir in the soft cheese, Cheddar and half the Parmesan. Leave for the cheese to melt into the sauce for a few minutes and stir.

- Now you are ready to layer up your lasagne in a large baking dish.

- Preheat the oven to 200°C/180°C fan/400°F/Gas mark 6.

- This lasagne has 3 layers so you need to use a third of the ingredients each time. Layer up in the order of meat sauce, thin layer of courgette, then cheese sauce. Do this 3 times, finishing with cheese sauce and topping with the rest of the Parmesan.

- Bake in the oven for 30–40 minutes until golden and bubbling.

Autumn vegetable crumble

327 calories

This is a super healthy and filling vegetarian meal.

Serves 4   Preparation time: 10 minutes   Cook time: 1 hour 25 minutes

Vegetarian

2 tbsp olive oil (198 cals)
1 large onion, peeled and chopped (86 cals)
2 garlic cloves, peeled and sliced (6 cals)
1 red chilli, deseeded and chopped (3 cals)
1 × 400g (14oz) can chopped tomatoes (64 cals)
300ml (1¼ cups) white wine (198 cals)
500ml (generous 2 cups) vegetable stock (35 cals)
1 bay leaf
2 fresh thyme sprigs (or ½ tsp dried)
600g (1¼lb) butternut squash (about 1 large), peeled, deseeded and cut into chunks (216 cals)
1 × 400g (14oz) can butter (lima) beans, rinsed and drained (220 cals)
50g (⅓ cup) wholemeal (wholewheat) breadcrumbs (108 cals)
5g (1 tsp) Parmesan, grated (21 cals)
25g (generous ⅛ cup) chopped nuts (152 cals)
handful of fresh parsley (10g/⅓oz), chopped (3 cals)
Salt and freshly ground black pepper

continued

- Heat 1 tablespoon of oil in a large pan, add the onion and fry gently for 8 minutes. Add the garlic and chilli and fry for a further 2 minutes.
- Stir in the chopped tomatoes, white wine, vegetable stock, bay leaf and thyme. Bring to the boil, then reduce the heat to medium–low and simmer, uncovered, for 20 minutes.
- Add the butternut squash and cook for a further 20 minutes. Stir in the butter (lima) beans.
- Preheat the oven 180°C/160°C fan/350°F/Gas mark 4.
- Mix the breadcrumbs, Parmesan, chopped nuts, parsley and the remaining tablespoon of oil together.
- Transfer the vegetable sauce to a suitable casserole dish and sprinkle on the crumble topping. Season liberally with salt and pepper. Bake in the oven for 30 minutes or until the crumble is golden and crisp.

WINTER

WINTER RECIPES

Under 200 calories

Moroccan spiced eggs

Porridge with cinnamon sugar

Hearty root vegetable soup

Borscht (chunky beetroot soup)

Savoy cabbage and Stilton soup

Slow onion soup

Warm lentil and leek salad

Traditional red cabbage with apple

Winter veg with onion gravy

Lemon meringue fool

Mini chocolate pear pie

Dark chocolate soufflé

Under 300 calories

All-in-one breakfast

Vegetarian breakfast

Mexican bean soup

Leek 'pasta' with cheesy mushroom sauce

Mixed bean chilli

Celeriac and white bean mash

Guilt-free cauliflower crust pizza

Red Thai veg curry
Fusion chicken thighs
Grainy mustard and honey chicken
Turkey meatballs with vegetable noodles
Turkey and almond stir-fry
Sticky pork with apple
Quick Italian beef stew
Beef and celeriac gratin
Fruit and seed flapjacks

Under 400 calories

Baked mushroom and blue cheese risotto
Parsnip and leek frittata
Tinned salmon and bean 'salad'
Chicken tikka masala
Chicken, rice and peas
Lamb pot roast
Traditional goulash
Beef bourguignon

MAKE NEW YEAR'S RESOLUTIONS AND STICK TO THEM

Ah, the dark days of winter. The cold can get to your bones – when you are dieting especially. Make sure your environment is warm. Sit by the radiator; wear lots of layers; even wear fingerless gloves while typing – I have done it!

There is one obvious aid for the winter fast day blues – and that is soup, and lots of it! A hearty winter soup will warm the cockles like nothing else can. Make a batch at the weekend and it will last over several diet days. You could even freeze some and then mix and match. Here you will find plenty of filling meat, stew and curry recipes – all designed to fill you up and beat off the cold.

If you are reading this in the bleak light of January, a few days after making a New Year's resolution, then take comfort in the thought that you are not alone. In fact this is the most popular time to start a diet and the gyms are buzzing. Here's how to make sure that YOUR story is a success. A simple and doable lifestyle change really is the best. So if your mission is to lose weight using the 2-Day Diet then you have chosen well: the diet has real, sustainable results. Prepare yourself well for your diet days, by shopping and preparing your food in advance.

Mid-winter may not the easiest time of year to start a diet, so set yourself some goals. You have probably got six months before the summer holidays hit. So use this time to prepare, prepare, prepare. Have you got a set target weight to lose? Be realistic but also celebrate every time you hit a goal: be it large or small.

A lot of the winter food is very filling and sustaining. Try the simple Celeriac and white bean mash (see page 196) for a quick winter's day filler. I also love hot and spicy food over the winter – the Mixed bean chilli (see page 195) is very tasty (and freezer-friendly). If you want an easy, warming dinner then you can't beat the Chicken tikka masala (see page 214).

Menu plans for diet days

Use these planners to inspire your cooking on diet days. It's amazing how much good food you can eat for under 500–600 calories.

Just work out whether you want three small meals/breakfast and dinner/lunch and dinner on your diet days and choose the right planner for you. If you need more help working out which plan is right for you have a look at *What kind of dieter are you?* (see page 6).

Feel free to swap a recipe for another with a similar calorie content if necessary.

MENU PLANS FOR DIET DAYS: WOMEN (WINTER)

WOMEN: 3 SMALL MEALS

	Breakfast	Lunch	Dinner	Cals
Day 1	Porridge with cinnamon sugar (page 180) 173 cals	Traditional red cabbage with apple (page 186) 79 cals	Grainy mustard and honey chicken (page 201) 244 cals	496
Day 2	Moroccan spiced eggs (page 179) 155 cals	Hearty root vegetable soup (page 181) 100 cals	Sticky pork with apple (page 206) 242 cals	497

WOMEN: BREAKFAST AND DINNER

	Breakfast	Dinner	Cals
Day 1	All-in-one breakfast (page 191) 270 cals	Celeriac and white bean mash (page 196) 231 cals	501
Day 2	Porridge with cinnamon sugar (page 180) 173 cals	Red Thai veg curry (page 199) (263) 100g (3½oz) Saffron 'rice' cauliflower (page 48) (34) 297 cals	470

	Lunch	Dinner	Cals
WOMEN: LUNCH AND DINNER			
Day 1	Savoy cabbage and Stilton soup (page 183) *171 cals*	Traditional goulash (page 218) *324 cals*	**495**
Day 2	Winter veg with onion gravy (page 187) *166 cals*	Tinned salmon and bean 'salad' (page 213) *334 cals*	**500**

MENU PLANS FOR DIET DAYS: MEN (WINTER)

	Breakfast	Lunch	Dinner	Cals
MEN: 3 SMALL MEALS				
Day 1	All-in-one breakfast (page 191) *270 cals*	Hearty root vegetable soup (page 181) *100 cals*	Quick Italian beef stew (page 207) *229 cals*	**599**
Day 2	Porridge with cinnamon sugar (page 180) *173 cals*	Winter veg with onion gravy (page 187) *166 cals*	Turkey and almond stir-fry (page 205) *254 cals*	**593**

MEN: BREAKFAST AND DINNER

	Breakfast	Dinner	Cals
Day 1	Vegetarian breakfast (page 192) 289 cals	Baked mushroom and blue cheese risotto (page 211) 304 cals	593
Day 2	All-in-one breakfast (page 191) 270 cals	Tinned salmon and bean 'salad' (page 213) 334 cals	604

MEN: LUNCH AND DINNER

	Lunch	Dinner	Cals
Day 1	Mexican bean soup (page 192) 218 cals	Sticky pork with apple (page 206) (242) 40g (scant ¼ cup) brown rice (143) 385 cals	603
Day 2	Winter veg with onion gravy (page 187) 166 cals	Chicken, rice and peas (page 216) 399 cals	565

WINTER RECIPES

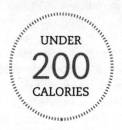

Moroccan spiced eggs

155 calories

This unusual dish is great served for breakfast/lunch or even brunch. You can make the tomato sauce first and reheat it when you are ready to cook the eggs.

Serves 2   Preparation time: 10 minutes   Cook time: 50 minutes

Vegetarian

1 tsp olive oil (27 cals)
1 garlic clove, peeled and finely chopped (3 cals)
1 tbsp tomato purée (30 cals)
¼ tsp cayenne pepper (4 cals)
¼ tsp ground cinnamon
¼ tsp ground cumin
pinch of salt
1 × 400g (14oz) can chopped tomatoes (64 cals)
small handful of flat-leaf (Italian) parsley (10g/⅓oz), chopped (3 cals)
2 large eggs at room temperature (178 cals)

continued

- Heat the oil in a small lidded saucepan, add the garlic and fry gently for 1 minute until just starting to brown. Add the tomato purée (paste), spices and salt. Continue to fry for a further 1–2 minutes. Add the chopped tomatoes and increase the heat to medium. With the lid off the pan, simmer the sauce for 30 minutes – make sure it is gently bubbling throughout and it should reduce in volume by about one-third.

- Reduce the heat to a minimum and stir in the chopped parsley. When you are ready to cook the eggs, crack them on the side of the saucepan and lower them gently into the tomato sauce. Put the lid on the pan and cook for 15 minutes (check after 10 minutes). Serve the concoction in individual bowls with the eggs floating on the top.

Porridge with cinnamon sugar

173 calories

Adding cinnamon provides a little extra sweetness without adding to the calories.

Serves 1   Preparation time: 2 minutes   Cook time: 5 minutes

30g (⅓ cup) porridge (rolled) oats (107 cals)
150ml (⅔ cup) skimmed (skim) milk (48 cals)
1 tsp muscovado (soft brown) sugar (18 cals)
¼ tsp ground cinnamon

- Place the oats, milk and 75ml (⅓ cup) water in a small saucepan and heat over a high heat until just boiling. Reduce the heat to a simmer and cook gently, stirring frequently, for about 5 minutes. When cooked it should be thick but not too sticky.

- Mix the sugar and cinnamon together in a small cup. You could make a batch of this to last several days.

- Serve the porridge in a small bowl with the cinnamon sugar sprinkled over.

Hearty root vegetable soup

100 calories

You can't get anything more warming and filling for 100 calories.

Serves 4   Preparation time: 10 minutes   Cook time: 25 minutes
Freezer-friendly

1 potato (170g) (128 cals)
2 medium carrots (70 cals)
1 small swede (rutabaga), about 300g (11oz) (72 cals)
1 turnip (80g/3oz) (18 cals)
1 medium parsnip (80g/3oz) (51 cals)
1 leek, trimmed and sliced (26 cals)
500ml (generous 2 cups) vegetable stock (fresh or made with 1 cube) (35 cals)
salt and freshly ground black pepper

- Peel and roughly chop the root vegetables.
- Place all the vegetables and the stock in a large saucepan and bring to the boil. Put the lid on, reduce the heat and simmer gently for 20 minutes.
- Blend in a blender or food processor until smooth, then return the soup to the pan and reheat gently, adding a little water if it is too thick.
- Season generously to taste and serve.

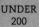
Borscht (chunky beetroot soup)

134 calories

This is a Russian soup and I have left it chunky in the Russian style, but you could purée it if you prefer. I use a vacuum pack of cooked beetroot for simplicity, making sure they are in natural juices not vinegar.

Serves 4   Preparation time: 5 minutes   Cook time: 25 minutes

Vegetarian, freezer-friendly

1 tbsp sunflower oil (99 cals)

1 carrot, peeled and chopped (35 cals)

1 medium onion, peeled and chopped (54 cals)

1 celery stick, trimmed and chopped (5 cals)

1 small parsnip (60g/2¼oz), peeled and chopped (38 cals)

1 litre (4 cups) vegetable stock (fresh is best but
you could use 2 cubes) (70 cals)

8 small beetroot (500g/1lb 2oz), cooked, chopped
into large chunks (230 cals)

juice of ½ lemon (2 cals)

freshly ground black pepper

- Heat the oil in a large lidded saucepan over a low heat, add the carrot, onion, celery and parsnip, then stir and put the lid on. Allow the vegetables to sweat for 10 minutes.
- Add the stock, bring to the boil, then reduce the heat and simmer with the lid off for 10 minutes. Add the beetroot and simmer for another 5 minutes.
- Add the lemon juice and pepper to taste.

Savoy cabbage and Stilton soup

171 calories

Serves 4   Preparation time: 10 minutes   Cook time: 30 minutes

Vegetarian, freezer-friendly

1 tsp olive oil (27 cals)
2 leeks, trimmed and sliced (53 cals)
1 potato (170g/6oz), peeled and diced (128 cals)
250ml (generous 1 cup) vegetable stock, fresh or made with ½ cube (18 cals)
¼ Savoy cabbage (100g/3½oz), outer leaves removed and shredded (27 cals)
50g (⅓ cup) Stilton, crumbled (205 cals)
2 tbsp sherry (28 cals)
200ml (generous ¾ cup) skimmed (skim) milk (64 cals)
2 tbsp (30ml) double (heavy) cream (135 cals)
salt and freshly ground black pepper

- Heat the oil in a large saucepan and gently fry the leeks for 10 minutes until tender.
- Stir in the potato and add the stock. Bring to the boil, then reduce the heat and simmer gently for 15 minutes. Use a potato masher in the soup to mash the potatoes until smooth (or blend in a blender if you prefer).
- Add the cabbage, Stilton, sherry, milk and cream. Bring to a gentle simmer and cook for 5 minutes until the cabbage is tender. Season well before serving.

Slow onion soup

197 calories

You need to cook the onions long and slow to get that beautiful onion sweetness.

Serves 4   Preparation time: 10 minutes   Cook time: 1 hour 30 minutes

Freezer-friendly

1 tbsp olive oil (99 cals)
15g (1 tbsp) butter (112 cals)
1kg (2¼lb) onions, peeled and finely sliced (360 cals)
1 garlic clove, peeled and finely sliced (3 cals)
2 fresh thyme leaves, finely chopped (or 1 tsp dried thyme)
1 bay leaf
salt and freshly ground black pepper
150ml (⅔ cup) red wine (129 cals)
1.2 litres (5 cups) beef stock (fresh is really good here, but can use 2 cubes) (70 cals)
1 tsp caster sugar (16 cals)

- Heat the oil and butter gently in a wide lidded frying pan (skillet). When the butter has melted, add the onions, garlic, thyme and bay leaf. Season generously with salt and pepper and stir.
- With the heat on the lowest possible setting, put the lid on the pan and cook for about 1 hour, stirring occasionally.
- Add the wine, stock and sugar, then bring to the boil, reduce the heat and simmer for 30 minutes before serving.

Warm lentil and leek salad

156 calories

So simple and filling.

Serves 2   Preparation time: 5 minutes   Cook time: 12 minutes

Vegetarian, quick & easy

2 leeks, trimmed and sliced (53 cals)

....

1 × 400g (14oz) can cooked Puy lentils, rinsed
and drained (172 cals)

....

100g (3½oz) baby spinach leaves (25 cals)

For the dressing:

2 tsp extra virgin olive oil (54 cals)

....

2 tsp red wine vinegar (1 cal)

....

¼ tsp English mustard (3 cals)

....

pinch of sugar (4 cals)

....

½ tsp dried mixed herbs

....

salt and freshly ground black pepper

....

- Place the leeks in a lidded saucepan together with about 50ml (scant ¼ cup) water. Put the lid on the pan and cook gently for about 10 minutes or until the leeks are just tender.
- Meanwhile, combine all the dressing ingredients together in a small bowl.
- Stir the Puy lentils into the leeks and cook for a further 2 minutes. Add the spinach leaves and stir in. Remove from the heat and stir in the dressing. Serve immediately.

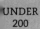
Traditional red cabbage with apple

79 calories

No one seems to cook red cabbage any more. It's easy to do, sweet and filling, and makes a great low-calorie accompaniment to red meat or stews. What's more it will keep in the fridge for up to a week and can be served hot or cold.

Serves 4   Preparation time: 10 minutes   Cook time: 55 minutes

Vegetarian, slow cooking

1 tsp olive oil (27 cals)
½ medium onion, peeled and chopped (17 cals)
1 garlic clove, peeled and chopped (3 cals)
1 tbsp caraway seeds, optional but good!
1 medium red cabbage (about 800g/1¾lb), quartered, cored and sliced (168 cals)
2 apples, peeled, cored and cut into eighths (94 cals)
juice and zest of ½ lemon (2 cals)
1 tsp balsamic vinegar (5 cals)
salt and freshly ground black pepper

- Heat the olive oil in a large lidded saucepan over a medium heat and fry the onion for 5 minutes until soft and lightly caramelized. Add the garlic and caraway seeds and cook for 30 seconds or until the seeds start to pop.
- Add the rest of the ingredients with 100ml (scant ½ cup) water, put the lid on, reduce the heat to low and cook for 45 minutes or until tender. Stir and check the water levels once or twice during cooking. If there's still a little water left in the pan at the end of the cooking time, remove the lid and cook for another 5 minutes.
- The red cabbage can also be slow cooked in a low oven or slow cooker on low for 4–6 hours.

Winter veg with onion gravy

166 calories

This is a great way to use up whatever winter vegetables you have around. Feel free to chop and change on the veg you use.

Serves 2   Preparation time: 10 minutes   Cook time: 40 minutes

1 carrot, peeled and roughly chopped (35 cals)

½ swede (rutabaga) (200g/7oz) or 2 turnips, peeled
and roughly chopped (48 cals)

1 medium parsnip, peeled and roughly chopped (64 cals)

1 tbsp sunflower oil (99 cals)

salt and freshly ground black pepper

1 onion, peeled and cut into half rings (54 cals)

250ml (generous 1 cup) beef stock (fresh or made
from 1 cube) (18 cals)

1 tsp English mustard (11 cals)

½ tsp Worcestershire sauce (2 cals)

- Preheat the oven to 200°C/180°C fan/400°F/Gas mark 6.
- Put the chopped carrot, swede (rutabaga) or turnips and parsnip on a baking tray and pour on two-thirds of the oil (reserving about a teaspoon in a frying pan/skillet for the onions). Toss the oil through the vegetables – this is easiest by hand – so that the vegetables are evenly coated. Season generously with salt and pepper, then pop into the oven and roast for about 30 minutes.
- Put the remaining oil into a wide lidded frying pan (skillet) and add the onion. When the onions start to sizzle give them a stir and turn the heat to the lowest setting. Put the lid on and let the onions cook slowly for 15–20 minutes until soft and brown, stirring occasionally.
- Add the stock, mustard and Worcestershire sauce to the onions, stir and bring to a gentle simmer. Cook for a further 10 minutes and serve over the roasted vegetables.

Lemon meringue fool

127 calories

A little lemony treat that is easy to whip up.

Serves 2   Preparation time: 5 minutes

Quick & easy

juice of ½ lemon (2 cals)
2 tbsp (30g/1¼oz) lemon curd (85 cals)
200g (generous ¾ cup) 0% fat Greek yogurt (114 cals)
1 meringue nest (52 cals)
lemon zest, to decorate

- Combine the lemon juice with the lemon curd.
- Place the Greek yogurt in a bowl and fold in the lemon curd. Do not overmix, you want them to be only just combined.
- Crumble the meringue into the lemon yogurt, reserving a few crumbs for the top. Fold the meringue in gently.
- Transfer the fool to 2 dishes or glasses. Top with the remaining meringue and a little lemon zest.

Mini chocolate pear pie

181 calories

This fab little chocolate pudding will brighten up any mealtime. Serve warm or cool and refrigerate for up to two days.

Serves 4   Preparation time: 20 minutes   Cook time: 40 minutes

4 pears, peeled, cored and chopped into small pieces (240 cals)
juice of ½ lemon (2 cals)
2 tsp soft light brown sugar (36 cals)
1 tbsp brandy (34 cals)
50g (scant ½ cup) icing (confectioners') sugar (196 cals)
1 tbsp (unsweetened) cocoa powder (47 cals)
25g (¼ cup) ground almonds (153 cals)
1 large egg, white only (18 cals for egg white)

- Preheat the oven to 160°C/140°C fan/325°F/Gas mark 3.
- Put the pears in a saucepan with the lemon juice, brown sugar, brandy and 3 tablespoons water. Bring to the boil, reduce the heat and cook, covered, for 10 minutes. Uncover, turn the heat up and cook for a further 5 minutes until the sauce has thickened.
- Spoon the pears and sauce into 4 ramekins.
- Mix the icing (confectioners') sugar, cocoa and ground almonds together in a bowl.
- In a clean bowl, whisk the egg white until it forms peaks, then fold (not mix) into the dry ingredients. Spoon over the pears and shake to level the mixture.
- Bake in the oven for 20 minutes.

Dark chocolate soufflé

195 calories

For when you need a chocolate hit! These lovely pots of chocolate can be frozen before cooking and then cooked from frozen in 12 minutes.

Serves 6   Preparation time: 20 minutes   Cook time: 10 minutes

Freezer-friendly

½ tsp sunflower oil (14 cals)

100g (3½oz/3½ squares) 70% dark chocolate (510 cals)

2 large eggs, separated (182 cals)

100g (½ cup) caster (superfine) sugar (394 cals)

4 medium eggs (egg whites only) (72 cals)

pinch of salt

- Preheat the oven to 210°C/190°C fan/400°F/Gas mark 6.
- Using kitchen paper (paper towels), lightly wipe the oil around the inside of 6 ramekins.
- Break the chocolate into pieces and place in a heatproof bowl. Place the bowl over a pan of gently simmering water, making sure the bowl doesn't touch the water. As soon as the chocolate has melted, remove from the heat.
- Whisk together the 2 egg yolks with half the sugar. This is much easier with an electric whisk. Continue beating until it becomes pale and thick. Stir in the melted chocolate.
- Wash the beaters with hot soapy water and dry thoroughly – this, together with a clean bowl, is necessary for stiff egg whites.
- Whisk the 6 eggs whites with the remaining sugar until it forms stiff peaks.
- Fold half the egg whites into the chocolate mixture and stir lightly with a metal spoon. Fold in the rest of the egg whites.
- Divide the soufflé mixture between the ramekins and place on a baking tray. Bake in the oven for 10 minutes (12 minutes from frozen) until puffed up.
- Serve immediately.

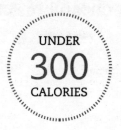

UNDER
300
CALORIES

All-in-one breakfast

270 calories

This one-pan breakfast is a great way to start a fast day.

Serves 1   Preparation time: 10 minutes   Cook time: 20 minutes

Quick & easy

1 good-quality sausage (50g/1¾oz) (154 calories)
100g (3½oz) mushrooms, sliced (13 cals)
1 medium tomato, halved (14 cals)
1 large egg, beaten (89 cals)

- Put your frying pan (skillet) over a medium heat. When hot, add the sausage and cook, turning every 1–2 minutes, for 12 minutes until browned on all sides.
- Add the mushrooms to the pan and fry in the sausage fat for about 3 minutes until browned. Push your mushrooms and sausage to the side, add the tomato, face down, and fry for 2 minutes.
- Turn the tomatoes over and move to the side and turn the heat to low. Pour the egg into the gap and fry slowly, stirring often, until scrambled but still soft. Serve immediately.

Vegetarian breakfast

289 calories

Serves 1   Preparation time: 5 minutes   Cook time: 10 minutes

Vegetarian, extra filling, quick & easy

1 tsp sunflower oil (27 cals)
....
100g (3½oz) mushrooms, sliced (13 cals)
....
1 medium tomato, halved (14 cals)
....
200g (7oz) reduced sugar and salt baked beans (146 cals)
....
1 large egg, beaten (89 cals)
....

- Heat the oil in a wide frying pan (skillet) over a medium–high heat. When hot, toss in the mushrooms and fry for 3 minutes until golden all over.
- Push the mushrooms to the side and put the tomato in the pan face down. Fry for 2 more minutes. Turn the heat to low, turn the tomato over and push to the side. Add the baked beans and warm through for a few minutes.
- Finally, make space for the egg and fry slowly, stirring often, until scrambled but still soft. Serve immediately.

Mexican bean soup

218 calories

Feel free to use any beans you like here. Or if you use dried beans, follow the packet instructions for soaking, boil the soup hard for 10 minutes and simmer for about an hour.

Serves 4   Preparation time: 10 minutes   Cook time: 1 hour

Vegetarian, extra filling, freezer-friendly

continued

1 tbsp sunflower oil (99 cals)
1 onion, peeled and finely chopped (54 cals)
2 celery sticks, trimmed and finely chopped (10 cals)
1 carrot, peeled and finely chopped (35 cals)
3 garlic cloves, peeled and finely chopped (9 cals)
2 red chillies, peeled, deseeded and chopped (4 cals)
2 bay leaves
1 fresh thyme and/or rosemary sprig
1 × 400g (14oz) can black-eyed peas (281 cals)
1 × 400g (14oz) can kidney beans (210 cals)
2 × 400g (14oz) cans chopped tomatoes (128 cals)
1 tbsp cumin seeds (or 1 tsp ground cumin)
2 tsp dried oregano (6 cals)
2 tbsp dry sherry or similar (28 cals)
juice of 2 limes (8 cals)
handful of fresh coriander (cilantro), chopped (optional)
salt and freshly ground black pepper

- Heat the oil in a large lidded pan over a low heat. Add the onion, celery, carrot, garlic, chillies, bay leaves and thyme or rosemary. Put the lid on the pan and cook gently for 15 minutes until tender.
- Add the beans, tomatoes, cumin, oregano and sherry and simmer for 30–40 minutes, stirring occasionally. Crush some of the beans with the back of the spoon and stir in – this will thicken the soup.
- Finally, add the lime juice and coriander (cilantro). Season generously and serve.

Leek 'pasta' with cheesy mushroom sauce

261 calories

I love this recipe as it's easy to cook for one. I use leeks to make the base of the recipe and it makes strands rather like short tagliatelle. You could also substitute the Parmesan for Cheddar – it has a similar amount of calories – just make sure you don't use too much!

Serves 1   Preparation time: 10 minutes   Cook time: 15 minutes

Quick & easy

3 medium or 2 large leeks (360 g) (79 cals)
1 tsp olive oil (27 cals)
250g (9oz) mushrooms, sliced (32 cals)
1 tbsp light soft cheese (55 cals)
15g (⅛ cup) fresh Parmesan, finely grated (68 cals)
freshly ground black pepper

- Trim the leeks, then make a deep cut down the long side of the leek that goes right to the centre. Wash each leek by opening up the leek under running water and rubbing out any dirt. Squeeze the leek after washing to remove any excess water. Cut the leeks into ribbons about 5mm (¼in) wide.
- Heat the oil in a lidded frying pan (skillet) over medium-high heat. Once hot, add the leeks and fry for 5 minutes, stirring occasionally. Add the mushrooms and continue to fry for a further 2 minutes.
- Turn the heat to low, add 2 tablespoons water and put the lid on. Cook for 5 minutes.
- Remove the lid from the pan and stir in the soft cheese and half of the Parmesan. Add a little more water if necessary to loosen the sauce and heat for 1–2 minutes until gently bubbling.
- Transfer to a wide bowl and sprinkle over the remaining Parmesan and some black pepper. Serve immediately.

Mixed bean chilli

253 calories

A healthy version of a classic.

Serves 4   Preparation time: 10 minutes   Cook time: 1 hour 15 minutes
Vegetarian, extra filling, freezer-friendly, slow cooking

1 tsp olive oil (27 cals)

1 medium onion, peeled and chopped (54 cals)

1 green chilli, deseeded and finely chopped (1 cal)

1 red (bell) pepper, deseeded and finely chopped (45 cals)

2 garlic cloves, peeled and thinly sliced (6 cals)

¼ tsp chilli (red pepper) flakes

1 tsp mild chilli powder

½ tsp ground cumin

1 heaped tsp paprika (14 cals)

½ tsp (unsweetened) cocoa powder (3 cals)

salt and freshly ground black pepper

2 medium butternut squash (about 900g/2lb), peeled,
deseeded and roughly chopped (324 cals)

1 × 400g (14oz) can chopped tomatoes (64 cals)

1 × 400g (14oz) can kidney beans, rinsed and
drained (210 cals)

1 × 400g (14oz) can cannellini beans, rinsed and
drained (259 cals)

juice of 1 lime (4 cals)

continued

- In a large lidded casserole, heat the oil gently and add the onion, chilli, red (bell) pepper and garlic. Sweat gently with the lid on for about 10–15 minutes until tender.
- Add the spices, cocoa and salt and pepper and stir. Add the butternut squash and stir again.
- Next pour in the chopped tomatoes, both types of beans and top up with 400ml (1¾ cups) water – making sure all the ingredients are generously covered with the water.
- Bring to a simmer, cover and cook slowly for 1 hour.
- If you prefer you could cook in the oven at 190°C/170°C fan/375°F/ Gas mark 5 for 1 hour or in the slow cooker on low for 6–8 hours.
- Crush some of the butternut squash and/or beans with the back of the spoon to thicken the sauce. Stir in the lime juice and season to taste before serving.

Celeriac and white bean mash

231 calories

This tasty alternative to mashed potato is flavoursome and makes a really large and filling dish.

Serves 2   Preparation time: 5 minutes   Cook time: 25 minutes

Vegetarian, extra filling

½ medium celeriac, about 350g (12oz) peeled weight (63 cals)
....
salt and freshly ground black pepper
....
15g (1 level tbsp, watch out this isn't a lot!) butter (112 cals)
....
1 tbsp light soft cheese (55 cals)
....
1 tbsp wholegrain mustard (21 cals)
....
1 × 400g (14oz) can cannellini beans, drained and rinsed (210 cals)

continued

- Using a sharp knife, top and tail the celeriac and use the knife to remove the skin all round the outside. Be prepared to discard up to a quarter of the celeriac in the knobbly skin. Cut roughly into chunks and put in a large saucepan of cold salted water.
- Put the saucepan on to boil and cook the celeriac until soft. This will take approximately 25 minutes from cold.
- Drain the celeriac and return to the pan. Add the butter, soft cheese, mustard and salt and pepper and mash until smooth. Add the cannellini beans and mash again to rough consistency.
- Serve immediately.

Guilt-free cauliflower crust pizza

250 calories

If all you crave is a pizza then this is the way to do it on a fast day. It's pretty easy to do and practically guilt-free. Thank you to Lavender & Lovage for recipe inspiration.

Serves 2/makes 2 pizzas   Preparation time: 10 minutes

Cook time: 35 minutes

Vegetarian

½ head large cauliflower, cut into florets
(400g/14oz) (136 cals)

1 large egg (91 cals)

20g (4 tbsp) Parmesan cheese, finely grated (90 cals)

½ tsp dried mixed herbs

pinch of salt

1 tsp cornflour (cornstarch) (18 cals)

2 garlic cloves, peeled and crushed (6 cals)

2 tbsp (30g/1oz) passata (strained tomatoes) (11 cals)

continued

½ small red onion, peeled and thinly sliced (11 cals)
½ green (bell) pepper, deseeded and finely chopped (10 cals)
1 tsp olive oil (27 cals)
1 tsp balsamic vinegar (5 cals)
60g (2¼oz) low-fat mozzarella, sliced (95 cals)

- Preheat the oven to 210°C/190°C fan/400°F/Gas mark 6 and line a baking tray with baking parchment or a silicone sheet.
- Using a food processor reduce the cauliflower to fine grains, do not over-process as you do not want a purée. Place the cauliflower grains in a microwaveable bowl, cover with clingfilm (plastic wrap) and cook on high in the microwave for 5–6 minutes until tender.
- In a large mixing bowl combine the cauliflower, egg, Parmesan, herbs, salt, cornflour (cornstarch) and half the crushed garlic and mix well until you form a stiff dough.
- Divide the dough in half and press out the dough into 2 rough circles on the lined baking tray. Bake in the oven for 16–18 minutes.
- Meanwhile, prepare your toppings: mix the passata (strained tomatoes) with the remaining garlic and set aside. Place the red onion and green (bell) pepper, oil and vinegar in a microwaveable bowl, cover with clingfilm and cook on high in the microwave for 1–2 minutes.
- Smooth the garlic passata equally over both pizzas, top with the onion and peppers and finally finish with the mozzarella. Return to the oven and bake for a further 10 minutes or until the cheese bubbles.

Red Thai veg curry

263 calories

With the right combination of vegetables and flavours you really don't need any meat in this easy favourite.

Serves 2   Preparation time: 5 minutes   Cook time: 20 minutes

Vegetarian, quick & easy

60g (2 generous tablespoons/2¼oz)
Thai red curry paste (82 cals)

½ × 400ml (14fl oz) can reduced-fat coconut milk (146 cals)

1 medium butternut squash, about 450g (1lb),
peeled and roughly chopped (162 cals)

1 medium courgette (zucchini), trimmed and
roughly chopped (27 cals)

1 small aubergine (eggplant) (400g/14oz),
roughly chopped (60 cals)

1 red (bell) pepper, deseeded and roughly chopped (45 cals)

6–8 fresh basil leaves

juice of 1 lime (4 cals)

- Place the red curry paste in a large pan and fry gently for 2 minutes. Stir in the coconut milk and add the butternut squash, courgette (zucchini), aubergine (eggplant) and (bell) pepper. Add a little water if needed to cover the vegetables and cook for 15 minutes until tender.
- Stir in the lime juice and basil leaves before serving.

Fusion chicken thighs

214 calories

This brilliant one-pot recipe has flavours from all over the East. The pastes and purées make it really easy to put together. As this serves eight, I like to make a big batch and freeze it in smaller portions.

Serves 8   Preparation time: 15 minutes   Cook time: 4–7 hours

Freezer-friendly, slow cooking

2 tbsp Madras curry powder (56 cals)
8 skinless, boneless chicken thighs, about 720g (1lb 8oz) (785 cals)
1 tbsp sunflower oil (99 cals)
1 large onion, finely chopped (86 cals)
1 tbsp lemongrass paste (42 cals)
1 tbsp ginger paste (24 cals)
2 red chillies, deseeded and finely chopped (4 cals)
salt
8 kaffir lime leaves
10 curry leaves
250ml (generous 1 cup) carton coconut cream (490 cals)
1 tbsp tamarind paste (78 cals)
2 medium tomatoes, cut into eighths (29 cals)
1 tsp sugar (16 cals)

- Rub half the curry powder over the chicken thighs and set aside.
- Put the oil into a frying pan (skillet) and set over a medium–high heat. Add the onion and fry for 5 minutes until golden. Turn the heat to low and add the lemongrass, ginger paste, chillies, salt, remaining curry powder, lime leaves and curry leaves and fry for a further 3 minutes.

continued

- Place the chicken thighs in the base of a large casserole dish or slow cooker. Dollop the spice paste over the top and add 500ml (generous 2 cups) water.

In the oven
- Preheat the oven to 140°C/120°C fan/275°F/Gas mark 1 and cook for 2½ hours. Add the coconut cream, tamarind paste, tomatoes and sugar. Cook at the same temperature for a further hour.

In the slow cooker
- Cook for 5–6 hours on low in the slow cooker, then add the coconut cream, tamarind paste, tomatoes and sugar and cook for a further hour.

Grainy mustard and honey chicken

244 calories

This is a completely delicious meal in one pan.

Serves 2   Preparation time: 10 minutes   Cook time: 30 minutes

Quick & easy

200g (7oz) new potatoes (2–3 depending on size),
quartered (140 cals)

150g (5oz) green beans (36 cals)

1 tsp olive oil (27 cals)

2 skinless, boneless chicken thighs, about
180g (6½ oz) (196 cals)

salt and freshly ground black pepper

250ml (generous 1 cup) chicken stock (fresh or made
with ½ cube) (18 cals)

1 tsp cornflour (cornstarch), dissolved in a little
cold water (18 cals)

continued

1 tbsp wholegrain mustard (21 cals)

1 tsp honey (23 cals)

1 tsp balsamic vinegar (5 cals)

1 small handful of fresh parsley (10g/⅓oz),
chopped (3 cals)

- Place the potatoes in cold salted water and bring to the boil. The small potatoes should cook in about 12–15 minutes from cold. Add the green beans 3 minutes before the end of cooking time. Drain and return to the warm pan and put a lid on.

- Heat the oil in a wide deep frying pan (skillet) over a medium-high heat. Season the chicken thighs all over with salt and pepper and fry for 5–6 minutes on each side.

- Pour in the stock and bring to a simmer. Slowly stir in the cornflour (cornstarch) and allow to thicken. Cook at a brisk simmer for 5 minutes. Stir in the mustard, honey and vinegar.

- Add the potatoes and green beans to the pan and stir to coat. Heat through for 2 more minutes, then stir in the parsley before serving.

Turkey meatballs with vegetable noodles

276 calories

To make a good shape for the noodles in this recipe you need to use a good tool. My personal favourite is a julienne peeler as it is small and cheap. Alternatives are a mandoline or spiralizer. Don't worry if you don't have any of these things, the coarse side of a grater does a good job, but your noodles won't be as long.

Serves 2   Preparation time: 20 minutes   Cook time: 35 minutes

For the meatballs and sauce:

1 tsp olive oil (27 cals)

1 garlic clove, peeled and crushed (3 cals)

1 × 400g (14oz) can chopped tomatoes (64 cals)

1 bay leaf

few leaves of fresh basil, chopped

1 tsp red wine vinegar (1 cal)

250g (9oz) lean turkey breast mince
(ground turkey) (262 cals)

1 tsp cornflour (cornstarch) (18 cals)

1 large egg, white only (18 cals for egg white)

10g (2 tbsp) Parmesan cheese,
finely grated (45 cals)

½ tsp dried mixed herbs

few drops Worcestershire sauce (1 cal)

salt and freshly ground black pepper

continued

For the noodles:

1 tsp olive oil (27 cals)

1 medium carrot, peeled and cut into noodles (35 cals)

2 courgettes (zucchini), trimmed and cut into
noodles (54 cals)

- In a large, non-stick saucepan heat the oil gently. Stir in the garlic and fry for 1 minute before adding the chopped tomatoes, bay leaf, basil and vinegar. Bring to the boil, reduce the heat and simmer uncovered for 10 minutes.
- Meanwhile, make the meatballs. Put the turkey mince (ground turkey) in a large bowl. Add the cornflour (cornstarch), egg white, Parmesan, mixed herbs, Worcestershire sauce and salt and pepper. Using your hands, mix all the ingredients well, then form small meatballs about the size of a ping-pong ball. You should get 8–10 balls.
- Drop the meatballs into the sauce and spoon the sauce over them so they are covered. Cook for 20 minutes.
- To make the noodles, heat the oil in a wok or large frying pan (skillet) over a medium–high heat. When hot, stir in the carrot and stir-fry for 2 minutes. Add the courgettes (zucchini) and season well. Stir-fry for another 2 minutes until cooked yet firm.
- Divide the noodles between two bowls, and top with the meatballs and sauce.

Turkey and almond stir-fry

254 calories

A warming winter stir-fry.

Serves 2   Preparation time: 5 minutes   Cook time: 12 minutes

Quick & easy

1 tsp sunflower oil (27 cals)
1 medium onion, peeled and finely sliced (54 cals)
1 green (bell) pepper, deseeded and sliced (21 cals)
200g (7oz) diced turkey breast (210 cals)
200g (7oz) Savoy cabbage or spring greens, shredded (54 cals)
2 tbsp port (25 cals)
2 tsp cornflour (cornstarch) (36 cals)
1 tsp ground ginger (14 cals)
1 tbsp dark soy sauce (6 cals)
10g (2 tbsp/5 tsp) flaked (slivered) almonds (61 cals)

- Heat the oil in a wok or wide lidded frying pan (skillet) over a high heat. Add the onion and (bell) pepper and stir-fry for 2 minutes. Add the turkey and stir-fry for 4 minutes until browned.
- Stir in the cabbage and then reduce the heat to medium. Pour in 100ml (scant ½ cup) water and put the lid on the pan. Steam for about 4 minutes until the cabbage is just tender.
- Meanwhile, combine the port, cornflour (cornstarch), ginger and soy sauce in a small bowl.
- Remove the lid from the pan and stir in the port sauce. Stir-fry for 2–3 minutes until thick and glossy. Sprinkle the almonds over just before serving.

Sticky pork with apple

242 calories

Serves 2   Preparation time: 5 minutes   Cook time: 20 minutes

Quick & easy

1 tsp olive oil (27 cals)
2 × 100g (3½oz) lean pork steaks (294 cals)
1 shallot, peeled and very finely sliced (6 cals)
1 apple, cored and cut into eighths (52 cals)
1 garlic clove, peeled and crushed (3 cals)
1 tbsp maple syrup (79 cals)
2 tsp cider vinegar or white wine vinegar (2 cals)
1 tbsp wholegrain mustard (21 cals)

- Heat the oil in a large non-stick frying pan (skillet) over a medium–high heat. Add the pork and shallot and fry the pork for about 3–4 minutes on each side, until browned. Remove the pork from the pan and set aside to rest.
- Stir in the apple and turn the heat down to medium. Cook for a few minutes, until just starting to soften.
- Stir in the garlic, maple syrup, vinegar and 3 tablespoons water. Bring to the boil and return the pork to the pan. Spoon some of the liquid over the pork and cook gently for about 5 minutes or until the pork is cooked through.
- Stir in the mustard before serving.

Quick Italian beef stew

229 calories

Serves 2   Preparation time: 10 minutes   Cook time: 30 minutes

Quick & easy, freezer-friendly

1 tsp sunflower oil (27 cals)
200g (7oz) lean beef strips (246 cals)
salt and freshly ground black pepper
½ onion, peeled and sliced into half rings (27 cals)
1 garlic clove, peeled and thinly sliced (3 cals)
½ green (bell) pepper, deseeded and sliced (10 cals)
½ yellow (bell) pepper, deseeded and sliced (18 cals)
1 x 400g (14oz) can chopped tomatoes (64 cals)
½ tsp dried mixed herbs
a little fresh oregano (optional)
12 large black olives, pitted (62 cals)

- Heat the oil in a large pan over a high heat. Season the beef with salt and pepper. When the oil is hot, toss in the beef and stir-fry for 2 minutes. Remove the beef from the pan and set aside.
- Reduce the heat to medium and fry the onion, garlic and (bell) peppers for 5–10 minutes until tender. With the heat still at medium, add the tomatoes and herbs and simmer for 15 minutes.
- Stir through the beef strips and olives and heat for a further 2 minutes before serving.

Beef and celeriac gratin

282 calories

This recipe is made in two stages. You make a wine sauce and marinate the beef in the sauce overnight before assembling the pie. I promise you it is well worth the effort.

Serves 4   Preparation time: 15 minutes, plus marinating
Cook time: 2½ hours

1 tsp olive oil (27 cals)
1 large onion, peeled and finely chopped (86 cals)
1 celery stick, peeled and finely chopped (5 cals)
1 garlic clove, peeled and finely chopped (3 cals)
1 bay leaf
200ml (generous ¾ cup) red wine (172 cals)
400g (14oz) extra lean casserole beef steak (492 cals)
1 tbsp plain (all-purpose) flour (68 cals)
250g (9oz) mushrooms, sliced (32 cals)
1 tsp English mustard (11 cals)
500ml (generous 2 cups) beef stock (fresh or made from 1 cube) (35 cals)
1 small celeriac (about 500g/1lb 2oz peeled weight) (90 cals)
salt and freshly ground black pepper
50g (⅓ cup) wholemeal (wholewheat) breadcrumbs (108 cals)

continued

- Heat the oil in a frying pan (skillet) over a medium heat. Add the onion and celery and fry for 5 minutes. Add the garlic, bay leaf and red wine and bring to the boil. Reduce the heat and simmer for 10 minutes. Leave to cool.
- Place the beef in a wide bowl and pour the wine mixture over. Cover and refrigerate overnight or for at least 4 hours.
- Preheat the oven to 180°C/160°C fan/350°F/Gas mark 4.
- Put the marinated beef in the base of a large baking dish, together with the marinade. Sprinkle over the flour, then layer over the mushrooms.
- Stir the mustard into the beef stock and pour over the mushrooms. You want the mushrooms to be just covered but not swimming in the stock. Bake in the oven for 90 minutes.
- Meanwhile, prepare the celeriac. Half fill a large saucepan with cold salted water. Use a knife to top and tail the celeriac before trimming off the skin. Quarter the celeriac lengthways. Cut the celeriac into thin (about 5mm/¼in) slices – they should be vaguely triangular. Drop the celeriac slices into the saucepan of water. Bring to the boil, reduce the heat and simmer for 15–20 minutes until tender. Drain the celeriac and leave to cool.
- Remove the baking dish from the oven and layer half the celeriac on top, pushing the celeriac down gently into the beef sauce. Then add a final layer of celeriac and sprinkle on the breadcrumbs. Season with salt and pepper.
- Bake in the oven uncovered for 30–40 minutes until golden.

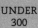

Fruit and seed flapjacks

247 calories per flapjack

These are a little bit naughty but very filling.

Makes 16 flapjacks   *Preparation time: 10 minutes*   *Cook time: 30 minutes*

Extra filling

175g (¾ cup) butter (1302 cals)
3 tbsp runny honey (259 cals)
150g (¾ cup) demerara (raw brown) sugar (591 cals)
100g (¾ cup) smooth peanut butter (607 cals)
225g (2⅔ cups) porridge (rolled) oats (801 cals)
50g (¼ cup) dried apricots, chopped (94 cals)
2 tbsp (20g/¾oz) sunflower seeds (116 cals)
2 tbsp sesame seeds (179 cals)

- Preheat the oven to 170°C/150°C fan/325°F/Gas mark 3. Line a 23cm (9in) square cake tin (pan) with 2 pieces of greaseproof paper. Arrange the paper in a cross shape so that all the sides are covered.
- Melt the butter, honey, sugar and peanut butter together in a pan over a low heat until the sugar has melted and everything is combined.
- Mix the oats, apricots and seeds together in a large bowl. Pour the melted butter mixture over and stir well.
- Press the mixture into the prepared tin and cook in the oven for 25–30 minutes until just starting to turn golden on top.
- Remove from the oven and leave to cool in the tin for about 10 minutes. Turn out onto a chopping (cutting) board and cut into 16 squares with a very sharp knife. Leave to cool completely on a wire rack. Store in an airtight container.

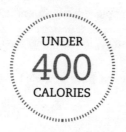

Baked mushroom and blue cheese risotto

304 calories

Baking the risotto in the oven makes this dish easy peasy. Just check the water levels a few times as you don't want it to dry out.

Serves 2   Preparation time: 10 minutes   Cook time: 1 hour

Vegetarian

1 tsp olive oil (27 cals)
1 red onion, peeled and chopped (54 cals)
200g (7oz) mushrooms, sliced (26 cals)
100g (½ cup) brown rice, rinsed (357 cals)
300ml (1¼ cups) vegetable stock (fresh or made with ½ cube) (18 cals)
juice of ½ lemon (2 cals)
30g (scant ¼ cup) blue cheese, crumbled (123 cals)
salt and freshly ground black pepper

- Preheat the oven to 200°C/180°C fan/400°F/Gas mark 6.
- Heat the oil in an ovenproof casserole, add the onion and fry for 3 minutes. Toss in the mushrooms and fry for a further 2 minutes.
- Tip in the rice and stir through. Add the stock and bring to a gentle simmer.

continued

- Cover with a lid and place in the oven. Cook for 45–55 minutes (reduce this to 20 minutes if you are using white rice), checking if you need to add more water halfway through, until the rice is tender.
- Stir through the lemon juice and blue cheese. Season to taste before serving.

Parsnip and leek frittata

348 calories

This is as good cold as hot, so keep the second half for your lunchbox tomorrow.

Serves 2   Preparation time: 10 minutes   Cook time: 30 minutes

Vegetarian

2 tsp olive oil (54 cals)
2 leeks, trimmed and chopped (52 cals)
2 medium parsnips, about 80g (3oz) each, peeled and roughly grated (102 cals)
3 large eggs (273 cals)
½ tsp English mustard (6 cals)
chopped fresh dill (optional)
50g (¼ cup) Pecorino cheese, grated (210 cals)
freshly ground black pepper

- In a lidded frying pan (skillet) heat half the oil over a medium–high heat. Toss in the leeks and grated parsnips and stir-fry for 2 minutes. Reduce the heat, add 2 tablespoons water and put the lid on. Sweat the leeks and parsnips for 10 minutes or until tender. Leave to cool.
- Put the eggs, mustard and dill in a bowl and whisk thoroughly. Stir in the grated cheese and cooled vegetables. *continued*

- Preheat the grill (broiler) to a medium setting.
- Choose a frying pan with a metal handle that can go under the grill. Wipe with kitchen paper (paper towels) dipped in the remaining oil. Heat over a medium–high heat and, when hot, add the egg mixture. Roll the pan around so the egg covers the base of the pan evenly. Immediately turn the heat to the lowest setting and cook, uncovered, for about 10 minutes or until the base and sides are firm.
- Sprinkle over the black pepper and put the pan under the grill for another 5–10 minutes until the top is firm and golden.
- Invert onto a plate. Serve immediately or leave to cool and serve in wedges.

Tinned salmon and bean 'salad'

334 calories

This is a fantastic 'storecupboard' salad. Although it serves two, I tend to make it just for me and refrigerate half. It keeps well in the fridge for up to two days and I think tastes even better the next day!

Serves 2   Preparation time: 10 minutes   Cook time: 5–8 minutes

Extra filling, quick & easy

100g (3½oz) green beans, fresh or frozen (24 cals)
½ red onion, peeled and cut into half rings (27 cals)
1 tbsp extra virgin olive oil (99 cals)
juice of 1 lemon (4 cals)
1 x 200g (7oz) can salmon (310 cals)
1 x 400g (14oz) can mixed beans, rinsed and drained (204 cals)
salt and freshly ground black pepper

continued

- Heat a small pan of water until boiling. Add the green beans and simmer for 3–4 minutes (fresh) or 5–6 minutes (frozen). Drain and leave to cool.

- Place the sliced onion in a small microwaveable bowl. Add the olive oil and lemon juice. Cover the bowl with clingfilm (plastic wrap) and microwave on high for 2 minutes. Leave to rest, covered, for a further 2 minutes.

- In a larger bowl, mix together the salmon, mixed beans and green beans. Pour the softened onion, oil and lemon juice over and combine. Season with salt and pepper. This can be served immediately or refrigerated in individual portions.

Chicken tikka masala

313 calories

While in no way authentic (and what is authentic for a chicken tikka masala anyway?) this a great way to cheer up a bleak winter's tea. It can be served on its own or with Saffron 'rice' cauliflower (page 48). This one-pot dish can be cooked in the oven in two hours or in a slow cooker for six hours.

Serves 4   Preparation time: 20 minutes   Cook time: 2–6 hours

Slow cooking, freezer-friendly

1 medium onion, peeled (54 cals)

2 garlic cloves, peeled (6 cals)

2cm (1in) piece of fresh ginger, peeled (10 cals)

1 tsp chilli (red pepper) flakes (or hot chilli powder)

2 heaped tsp paprika (28 cals)

½ tsp ground coriander

½ tsp ground cumin

½ tsp ground turmeric

continued

½ tsp dried mint (3 cals)

1 tsp salt

1 tbsp (20g) ground almonds (122 cals)

2 tbsp tomato purée (paste) (60 cals)

juice of 1 lime (4 cals)

2 tsp sunflower oil (54 cals)

200ml (generous ¾ cup) low-fat plain
yogurt (112 cals)

500g (1lb 2oz) skinless chicken breast, cut into
rough cubes (530 cals)

2 tbsp double (heavy) cream (269 cals)

- Preheat the oven to 140°C/120°C fan/275°F/Gas mark 1.
- Process the onion, garlic and ginger to a paste in a food processor or use a hand blender or grate using the large side of the grater for the onion and the fine side for the garlic and ginger. Either way they should be combined into a thick gloopy paste.
- Stir in the spices, mint, salt and ground almonds, then add the tomato purée (paste) and lime juice and mix well.
- Heat the oil in a frying pan (skillet) over a medium heat for 2 minutes before adding in the paste. It should sizzle nicely. Stir-fry for 1 minute until it starts to release its spicy aroma. Turn the heat down and stir in the yogurt and bubble gently for 1–2 minutes.
- Place the diced chicken in the base of a casserole dish or your slow cooker and pour the sauce over.
- Cook in the oven for 2 hours or in your slow cooker on low for 5–6 hours. Stir in the cream at the end of the cooking time.

Chicken, rice and peas

399 calories

This warming dish for one is a saviour on a cold winter's night. It's quick to cook and is so so satisfying.

Serves 1   Preparation time: 5 minutes   Cook time: 30 minutes

Extra filling

30g (scant ¼ cup) basmati rice (dry weight) (108 cals)
50g (scant ½ cup) frozen peas (33 cals)
few sprays of light oil spray (3 cals)
1 x 150g (5oz) skinless chicken breast, cut into strips (159 cals)
75ml (⅓ cup) skimmed (skim) milk (28 cals)
½ tbsp light soft cheese (27 cals)
10g (2 tbsp) mature (sharp) Cheddar, grated (41 cals)
salt and freshly ground black pepper

- Boil the rice as per the packet instructions. Add the frozen peas 6 minutes before the end of the cooking time. Drain and set aside.
- Heat the spray oil in a frying pan (skillet) over a medium heat and fry the chicken for 4–6 minutes, until browned all over and just cooked through.
- Add the milk, soft cheese and Cheddar to the frying pan. Bring to a gentle simmer and continue to cook gently for 5 minutes.
- Finally, add the cooked rice and peas to the pan and heat through. Season with salt and pepper.
- Serve immediately.

Lamb pot roast

367 calories

A warming and easy dish.

Serves 4   Preparation time: 10 minutes

Cook time: 2¼ hours–8¾ hours

Freezer-friendly, slow cooking

4 × 90g (3¼oz) lean lamb leg steaks (673 cals)
2 tsp turmeric
2 tsp English mustard (22 cals)
1 tsp sugar (16 cals)
salt and freshly ground black pepper
1 tbsp vegetable oil (99 cals)
1 medium onion, peeled and chopped (54 cals)
4 garlic cloves, peeled and chopped (12 cals)
1 medium sweet potato (about 130g), peeled and cut into large chunks (113 cals)
1 × 400g (14oz) can whole tomatoes (64 cals)
1 × 400g (14oz) can chickpeas, rinsed and drained (276 cals)
500ml (generous 2 cups) lamb or chicken stock (made from 1 stock cube) (35 cals)
100g (3½oz) spinach, fresh or frozen (about 4 cubes) (21 cals)
100g (scant 1 cup) peas, fresh (83 cals)

continued

- Rub the lamb all over with the turmeric, mustard, sugar and salt and pepper.
- In a casserole dish, heat the vegetable oil until it is smoking hot. Toss in the lamb and fry for 2 minutes each side. Reduce the heat and stir in the onion and garlic and fry gently for 2 minutes.
- Add the sweet potato, tomatoes, chickpeas and stock, then stir and put the lid on.

In the oven
- Preheat the oven to 180°C/160°C fan/350°F/Gas mark 4 and cook for 2 hours.
- Stir in the spinach and peas. Replace onto the hob, bring to a gentle simmer and cook for 10 minutes.

In the slow cooker
- Cook on low for 7–8 hours. Stir in the spinach and peas.
- Turn to high and cook uncovered for 30 minutes.

Traditional goulash

324 calories

This delicious Hungarian dish is a favourite in our household.

Serves 4   Preparation time: 20 minutes   Cook time: 2–9 hours

Freezer-friendly, slow cooking

400g (14oz) extra lean casserole beef steak, diced (492 cals)
1 tbsp plain (all-purpose) flour (68 cals)
salt and freshly ground black pepper
2 tbsp sunflower oil (198 cals)
1 large onion, chopped (86 cals)
2 garlic cloves, peeled and chopped (6 cals)
1 green (bell) pepper, deseeded and chopped (21 cals)

continued

| 1 red (bell) pepper, deseeded and chopped (45 cals) |
| 1 heaped tbsp paprika (42 cals) |
| 1 heaped tsp smoked paprika (14 cals) |
| 1 × 400g (14oz) can chopped tomatoes (64 cals) |
| 250ml (generous 1 cup) beef stock (fresh or made with ½ cube) (18 cals) |
| 150ml (⅔ cup) light crème fraîche (243 cals) |

- Sprinkle the beef with the flour and salt and pepper and toss until well coated.
- Heat the oil in a casserole dish over a high heat. Brown the steak in batches and set aside.
- Turn the heat to low and add the onion, garlic and (bell) peppers. Put the lid on and sweat until tender, about 10 minutes.
- Return the beef to the pan together with both types of paprika, the chopped tomatoes and beef stock. Bring to a simmer and cook with the lid off for 20–30 minutes.

On the hob
- Continue to cook over a low heat for about 1 hour, removing the lid towards the end of the cooking time.

In the oven
- Preheat the oven to 150°C/130°C fan/300°F/Gas mark 2 and cook for 3 hours.

In the slow cooker
- Transfer to a slow cooker and cook on low for 8 hours or overnight.

- Stir in the crème fraîche just before serving. The goulash freezes well and this can be done before or after the crème fraîche is added.

Beef bourguignon

359 calories

This is a very simple way to make an unauthentic but still very yummy bourguignon.

Serves 4   Preparation time: 10 minutes   Cook time: 3–8 hours

Freezer-friendly, slow cooking

400g (14oz) extra lean casserole beef steak, diced (492 cals)
100g (3½oz) lardons or bacon bits (276 cals)
200g (7oz) button mushrooms, washed (26 cals)
2 garlic cloves, peeled and sliced (6 cals)
1 medium onion, peeled, halved and sliced (54 cals)
200g (7oz) pickled shallots, drained (30 cals)
1 tsp dried thyme (3 cals)
2 bay leaves
2 tbsp plain (all-purpose) flour (204 cals)
salt and freshly ground black pepper
400ml (1¾ cups) red wine (344 cals)

- Put the beef, lardons, mushrooms, garlic, onion, shallots, thyme and bay leaves into a large casserole dish or slow cooker dish.
- Sprinkle on the flour and, using your hands, toss it around until everything is lightly coated in flour.
- Next, season with salt and pepper and pour on the wine and 100ml (scant ½ cup) water. Give it a stir and pop on the lid.

In the oven
- Preheat the oven to 140°C/120°C fan/275°F/Gas mark 1 and cook for 3 hours.

In the slow cooker
- Cook on low for 8 hours.
- Add a little water halfway through cooking if necessary.

SNACKS AND CHEATS

Snacks (under 100 calories)

Twenty guilt-free treats when you need a mini pick-me-up. Please note that average calorie counts have been given for generic foods (tomatoes, apples, eggs, etc.), but these will vary according to their individual size and weight.

Tasty veggies

1 medium carrot (100g/3½oz), cut into sticks	35 calories
1 red pepper, deseeded (160g/5¾oz), cut into sticks	51 calories
4 celery sticks (280g/10oz)	20 calories
10 cherry tomatoes	22 calories

Savoury delights

Babybel Light	63 calories
Large boiled egg	98 calories
1 tbsp reduced-fat houmous	27 calories

1 tbsp Old El Paso salsa	6 calories
1 Ryvita original	35 calories
1 tbsp light soft cheese (35g)	55 calories
Cup of soup	80–100 calories
(average value – check your own brand for confirmation)	
1 ready-to-eat Sharwood's poppadom	37 calories

Fruity favourites

1 apple (100g/3½oz)	47 calories
1 medium satsuma (70g/2½oz)	25 calories
10 grapes (50g/1¾oz)	30 calories

Sweet treats

Glass of skimmed milk (200ml/generous ¾ cup)	64 calories
Walls Mini Milk ice cream	30 calories
Cadbury hot chocolate Highlights	40 calories
3 squares 70% dark chocolate (10g/⅓oz)	51 calories
Müller light yogurt	90 calories

Feel free to mix and match

Carrot sticks from 1 carrot and reduced-fat houmous	62 calories
Babybel Light and 4 celery sticks	83 calories
Ryvita with 1 tbsp light soft cheese	90 calories

Plate fillers

If you have calculated your calories for a meal and have found you have a few to spare then this is the place to look. Generally if you have got 100 or more calories to play with then you could add some good carbohydrates, like rice or new potatoes. If you have got 50–100 calories to spare, consider adding a salad or mixed vegetables. And don't despair if you have got less than 50 calories left over, you can still have a plate full of carefully chosen green veg or salad leaves.

Ten 'good' carbohydrates

New potatoes go well with chicken or any dish with a sauce – 200g (7oz) new potatoes have 140 calories. That's about 4 small potatoes in their skins. Pop them on the scales to make sure you have the right amount.

Brown rice has a dense nutty flavour and is incredibly filling. A 40g (scant ¼ cup) portion (that's dry weight) has 143 calories. Note that brown rice takes about 30 minutes to cook – check the packet instructions. An easy alternative is precooked microwaveable brown rice. Try Tilda steamed microwave rice – half a 250g (9oz) packet has 158 calories.

Basmati rice is also a good carbohydrate and cooks in 10 minutes. I use a microwave rice cooker and it's a breeze. Again it is worth weighing the rice to make sure you get the correct amount. A 40g (scant ¼ cup) serving (dry weight) has 144 calories.

If you want a little extra crunch on the side of your plate, you could add an **oatcake** or two. Each oatcake has 62 calories. I like Nairns rough oatcakes.

Another crunchy plate addition is a **crispbread** such as Ryvita or Finn Crisp. An original Ryvita has 35 calories per slice and a

Finn Crisp has 45 calories per slice. There are loads of different variations on this theme, just check the side of the packet for individual calories.

Couscous is a great low-calorie grain. It's extremely easy to cook – just pour over boiling water, cover and leave to cook for about 10 minutes. A 40g (scant ¼ cup) (dry weight) portion has 91 calories.

Quinoa differs from other grains in that it mixes carbohydrate and protein. It is therefore particularly good with a vegetarian dish. You cook it similarly to rice and it takes about 15 minutes. A 40g (scant ¼ cup) dry weight serving has 124 calories.

Bulgur wheat makes an unusual addition to your plate. Cook according to the packet instructions (normally about 20 minutes). A 40g (scant ¼ cup) dry weight portion has 141 calories.

A small (150g/5oz) baked **sweet potato** has 130 calories. I find it easiest to microwave the sweet potato first for 3–4 minutes and then bake in a preheated oven at 200°C/180°C fan/400°F/Gas mark 6 for about 10 minutes. Don't forget to prick your sweet potato several times before cooking.

A slice of wholemeal (wholewheat) **bread** is perhaps the quickest addition to your plate. A medium slice from a sliced loaf has about 65 calories. Check the packet for the calorific content of your bread as it can vary considerably.

Salads, mixed vegetables and fruit

If you have got less than 100 calories to spare then consider a salad, mixed veg on the side OR a piece of fruit after. Please note that average calorie counts have been given for generic foods (tomatoes, apples, eggs, etc.), but these will vary according to their individual size and weight.

Salad 58 calories
1 Little Gem (Boston) lettuce, shredded *(20 cals)*
1 × 5cm (2in) piece cucumber, thinly sliced *(10 cals)*
2 medium tomatoes, sliced *(28 cals)*

Mixed veg 80 calories
1 carrot, peeled and sliced *(35 cals)*
50g (1¾oz) fine green beans *(12 cals)*
50g (1¾oz) frozen peas (frozen weight) *(33 cals)*

Fruit

Sometimes it's nice to leave yourself a few calories for a fruit 'treat' at the end of the meal. Here are some of my favourites.

1 small (80g/3oz) banana *(76 cals)*
1 medium orange (200g/7oz) *(52 cals)*
1 small satsuma (50g/1¾oz) *(18 cals)*
bunch of grapes (about 20/100g/3½oz) *(60 cals)*
100g (scant ¾ cup) strawberries *(27 cals)*
1 apple (100g/3½oz) *(47 cals)*

Very low-calorie vegetables

Some green vegetables and salad leaves are so low in calories that you can serve your meal with a plate full of veg and still only add a few calories. Try squeezing over the juice of ½ lemon (2 cals) or dribbling over 1 teaspoon of balsamic vinegar (5 cals) to bring out the best in the flavour.

100g (3½oz/about ½ head) broccoli *(33 cals)*
100g (3½oz) green beans *(24 cals)*
100g (3½oz) mangetout (snow peas) *(32 cals)*
50g (1¾oz) baby spinach *(12 cals)*/watercress *(11 cals)*/rocket (arugula) *(17 cals)*
80g (3oz) bag mixed leaf salad *(10–20 cals – check the packet to confirm)*

Flavour fixes

I never ever make bland food. If your dinner doesn't delight your taste buds then you are far more likely to want to eat something 'bad' afterwards.

There are many simple ways to do this without adding to the calories.

Salt and pepper

I know this sounds basic, but it makes such a difference that it is worth a special mention. I don't tend to include much salt while I am cooking but I always check the seasoning before I eat. Sometimes a little grind of salt will transform a dish. If you taste a sauce and you can't really taste any of the individual flavours then you may have under-salted. Add a little at a time, as oversalted food can be even worse. Likewise I don't think there are many dishes that are not enhanced by a little freshly ground black pepper sprinkled on at the end.

Herbs

Herbs are obviously great at making a fresh dish zing. I often find recipe books require you to have a fully stocked herb garden to make the most of their recipes and it is sometimes difficult to know which ones are essential and which ones are 'nice to have'.

My herb stocks are pretty basic and if I don't have the right herbs for the recipe then I just cook it anyway. The only dried herbs I have are mixed herbs and bay leaves. I pop a bay leaf into most meaty sauces and casseroles. I use the mixed herbs in place of any dried herbs a recipe suggests. Any sauce that is slow cooked (that's over 30 minutes) can benefit from dried herbs.

In terms of fresh herbs, I do love the flavour but I won't generally go out to the shops to buy a fresh herb even if a recipe claims that it's important. I have fresh mint in the garden (almost impossible to kill), but mint has a distinct taste and I only use this in dishes where I want a minty flavour. I also buy potted herbs from the supermarket, with basil and coriander (cilantro) being my favourites. If I remember to water them they can last for about a month and are much better value than the pre-cut ones. I add basil to any Italian-style dishes and salad dressings and I like to add a leaf or two right at the end of cooking. Fresh coriander is amazing in anything remotely spicy – Indian, Moroccan, Mexican and more. A bunch of fresh coriander, roughly chopped, really does enhance a dish, but, if I don't have any, it doesn't stop me cooking the recipe.

Onions and garlic

When you think about it, onions and garlic are ingredients you can't live without in most sauces and casseroles. Onions can be cooked slowly for a deep flavour – try sprinkling with a little salt to bring out their natural sweetness – or more quickly to get a caramelised golden onion with more bite. Cooking the onion slowly uses less oil or fat and it is generally good practice for sauces and casseroles. It tends to be used more often in low-calorie cooking. Garlic enhances the flavour of almost any sauce-based dish, and at only 4 calories a clove I like to use it liberally. If frying it should be added after the onion as it takes less time to cook. There are some recipes that benefit from fresh garlic, when it is used raw, for example, or when roasting.

TOP TIP! Try garlic purée in place of fresh garlic. I use it about 90 per cent of the time! This is because it is so much simpler and gives the flavour without the fuss. Use about 1 teaspoon (a squirt of about 2.5cm/1in if you use it from a tube) for each clove of garlic required. If frying, only fry for 1 minute as it can burn easily. I buy it in toothpaste-sized tubes, which keep for ages unopened and about six weeks in the fridge after opening.

Spice cupboard essentials

I love spicy food and have a drawer full of spices. These include the usual suspects plus a few really weird ones. If you are browsing through my recipes and think you'll never have all these – think again – there's only five or six essentials that are used time and time again. You should be able to find all these by the jar in the supermarket, or try a whole food shop where you may be able to buy them even cheaper by weight.

If you are new to spices then I would recommend investing in the following:

- paprika
- ground cumin
- turmeric
- chilli powder or chilli (red pepper) flakes
- ground ginger
- ground cinnamon

The only spices that are hot in this list are paprika and chilli powder. If you don't like your dishes too spicy, then you can buy mild versions of both of these. Ground ginger can be used as a substitute for fresh ginger. Follow the guideline quantities carefully as too much of a spice can ruin a dish. Cinnamon in particular can overpower everything else if you add too much.

You may also want to invest in some curry powder. A curry powder is just a blend of spices. If you don't have the right combination then you could just use this instead. A good one to choose would be a Madras or medium curry powder.

If you like things hot, then there are loads of different types of chillies, both fresh or dried, that you can use to add heat to your dishes in different ways. Chilli powder, cayenne pepper, chilli (red pepper) flakes or fresh chilli all provide heat to a recipe so you should feel free to vary these depending on your taste. Chilli powder normally comes in hot or mild varieties. If you don't like it too hot, stick to mild! If you want to be a bit of a curry connoisseur and you like it a bit hotter, try combining two types of heat for a more rounded and robust flavour. From hottest to mildest I would rate them as follows:

- Scotch bonnet fresh chilli with seeds
- bird's-eye fresh chilli with seeds
- cayenne pepper
- hot chilli powder
- chilli (red pepper) flakes
- standard fresh chilli, deseeded
- mild chilli powder

High calorie items and scales

There are a few items that really add to a dish, which I always keep on hand. I have to be very careful about how much I use as they are very calorific. They tend to be high fat and just don't have a low-calorie equivalent. For me, I think there are only four items on this list:

- butter (74 calories for 10g/2 tsp)
- chorizo (25–100 cals for 20g/¾oz – check the packet, as it varies considerably)
- Cheddar (82 calories for 20g/¾oz)
- Parmesan (42 calories for 10g/⅓oz)

They all have strong flavours and are used in some of my favourite dishes. With all of these ingredients, a little goes a long way and every gram or ounce counts. I would strongly recommend buying a set of digital scales. I use different scales from my standard kitchen scales, as kitchen scales are not accurate enough for weighing small quantities. These are available from hardware shops or from various online retailers. The best thing to search for is 'micro scales' and look for ones with an accuracy of up to 0.1g. They are very reasonably priced and you can calibrate most with a bowl on top OR weigh your food on a layer of clingfilm (plastic wrap).

Ten easy meals

Not got much time? Desperately hungry? Nothing in the fridge? Try these ten incredibly quick and easy dinners, all made from basic ingredients.

Beans on toast *212 calories*
1 × 200g (7oz) pot reduced sugar and salt beans *(147 cals)*
1 medium slice of wholemeal (wholewheat) bread *(65 cals)*

Omelette and salad *226 calories*
2 large eggs *(182 cals)*
80g (3oz) bag mixed leaf salad *(15 cals)*
5cm (2in) piece of cucumber, sliced *(10 cals)*
1 medium tomato *(14 cals)*
1 tsp balsamic vinegar *(5 cals)*

Fried chorizo with spinach *80 cals*
20g (¾oz) Spanish chorizo, thinly sliced and fried *(58 cals)*
2 spring onions (scallions), chopped *(10 cals)*
50g (1¾oz) baby spinach *(12 cals)*

Crispbread with cottage cheese and cucumber *138 cals*
2 crispbreads (such as Ryvita) *(70 cals)*
2 tbsp low-fat cottage cheese (80g/3oz) *(63 cals)*
4 slices cucumber *(5 cals)*

Fish fingers and salad 290 *cals*
3 fish fingers *(180 cals)*
1 Little Gem (Boston) lettuce *(20 cals)*
5cm (2in) piece of cucumber, sliced *(10 cals)*
10 cherry tomatoes *(22 cals)*
1 tbsp low-fat salad cream *(58 cals)*

'No carb' fry up 146 *calories*
1 slice of back (Canadian) bacon (20g/¾oz) *(43 cals)*
1 medium tomato, halved *(14 cals)*
100g (3½oz) mushrooms *(13 cals)*
1 egg, beaten *(76 cals)*

Garlic mushrooms 134 *cals*
1 tbsp olive oil *(99 cals)*
1 garlic clove, peeled and crushed *(3 cals)*
250g (9oz) mushrooms, sliced *(32 cals)*

Scrambled egg with tomato 217 *calories*
2 large eggs *(182 cals)*
1 tbsp semi-skimmed (skim) milk *(7 cals)*
2 medium tomatoes, chopped *(28 cals)*

Tinned tuna salad 192 *calories*
1 × 160g (5¾oz) can tuna in water, drained *(111 cals)*
80g (3oz) bag mixed leaf salad *(15 cals)*
2 medium tomatoes, sliced *(28 cals)*
1 gherkin or 2 cornichons, chopped *(5 cals)*
6 black olives *(31 cals)*
juice of ½ lemon *(2 cals)*

Cherry tomatoes with feta 158 *calories*
10 cherry tomatoes *(22 cals)*
50g (1¾oz) light feta cheese *(90 cals)*
¼ red onion, peeled and finely chopped *(14 cals)*
1 tsp extra virgin olive oil *(27 cals)*
1 tsp balsamic vinegar *(5 cals)*

Cheats

Sometimes we all need to cheat. Whether we are out and about and feel a bit wobbly or are staring at the shelves in the supermarket with zero desire to cook, we have all been there. So don't feel bad, just do it in style and don't break the calorie rules!

If you are looking for a light lunch

Avoid sandwiches, wraps, etc. and look at the salads. Anything without carbs will have a lot less calories. Salads made with fish such as tuna, crayfish or prawns (shrimp) are often really low calorie, even with dressing. A salad with beans or pulses may have slightly more calories but will fill you up and make you less likely to suffer from hunger pangs later on. Set your calorie limit for the meal and stick to it, no matter what other temptations you find. Beware of tasty extras and drinks that could easily double the calorie count of your meal.

For tasty and filling salads, Pret and M&S both have an excellent range.

If you are in a healthy fast food establishment

There are a few fast food chains now that make healthy claims. Generally you want to look for salads or soups without bread or noodles. A few restaurants include calorie counts on their menus and many include calorie counts on their websites, so it is worth checking before you choose.

I like **Leon** any day of the week. On a diet day I would tend to stick to soup, but I also like their Shredded kale & peanut salad, which has 244 calories with dressing.

Giraffe is also worth a look with a low-calorie egg white omelette and a different soup every day.

Finally, I find **Yo! Sushi** is a great place for a quick low-calorie lunch. All the food on the menu is calorie counted and there are plenty of items suitable for a diet day.

If you are in the supermarket

Any supermarket and most convenience stores will stock a 'diet' range with calorie counts attached. These can be a godsend if you are on your way home from work and need a quick, no fuss dinner. Plus the calorie counting is done for you, so you know exactly how many calories you have eaten. Of course all ready-meals have a sting in the tail, they are expensive and can be overloaded with salt. Diet ready-meals also have the disadvantage of giving you a much smaller portion than you might be expecting – this saves them money and helps them to keep the calorie count lower, but can leave you feeling dissatisfied.

I do think that the Marks & Spencer range is above average, with both their *Count on Us* and *Fuller Longer* ranges being suitable for diet days.

One of my favourite stand-bys is the Innocent Veg Pot (especially when they are on special offer!) I think the nutritional balance is good, and they are low calorie and also filling.

Finally, I believe steering away from the ready-meal section and looking at the fresh soups can be beneficial, although do check the portion sizes and calorie count as they can vary enormously.

CALORIE COUNTER

Food Type	cal per 100g/ml	pro (g)	carb (g)	fat (g)
Bread				
Breadcrumbs, manufactured	354	10.1	78.5	2.1
Brown bread	207	7.9	42.1	2
Brown, crusty	255	10.3	50.4	2.8
Brown, soft	236	9.9	44.8	3.2
Brown, toasted	272	10.4	56.5	2.1
Ciabatta	271	10.2	52	3.9
Currant bread	289	7.5	50.7	7.6
Garlic bread, prepacked, frozen	365	7.8	45	18.3
Granary	237	9.6	47.4	2.3
Granary, roll	238	10.2	42.7	4.2
Hamburger buns	264	9.1	48.8	5
Pitta, white	255	9.1	55.1	1.3
Tortillas, corn	222	6	47	3
White bread	219	7.9	46.1	1.6
White, crusty	262	9.2	54.9	2.2
White, soft	254	9.3	51.5	2.6
White, toasted	267	9.7	56.2	2
Wholemeal	217	9.4	42	2.5
Wholemeal breadcrumbs	217	9.4	42	2.5
Wholemeal, roll	244	10.4	46.1	3.3

Food Type	cal per 100g/ml	pro (g)	carb (g)	fat (g)
Wholemeal, toasted	255	11.2	49.2	2.9
Beans and Lentils				
Black-eyed peas (cooked)	116	8	21	1
Borlotti beans, canned and drained	53	4	6	1
Broad beans, raw	59	5.7	7.2	1
Butter beans (canned)	77	5.9	13	0.5
Cannellini beans, canned and drained	85	7.1	12.5	0.6
Chickpeas, canned and drained	115	7.2	16.1	2.9
Fine (green) beans	24	1.9	3.2	0.5
Mixed beans, canned	100	6	15	1
Puy lentils, cooked	105	8.8	16.9	0.7
Puy lentils, dried	297	24.3	48.8	1.9
Red kidney beans, canned and drained	100	6.9	17.8	0.6
Red lentils, split, dried	318	23.8	56.3	1.3
Breakfast Cereals				
Bran Flakes	330	10.2	71.2	2.5
Corn Flakes	376	7.9	89.6	0.9
Fruit 'n' Fibre	353	9	72.5	5
Muesli, Swiss style	363	9.8	72.2	5.9
Multi-Grain Start	369	7.9	85.2	3.5
Oat bran	325	10.6	67.7	3.5
Oat granola (homemade)	489	15	53	24
Porridge with water	46	1.4	8.1	1.1
Porridge with whole milk	113	4.8	12.6	5.1
Porridge (rolled) oats	356	11	60	8
Special K	374	15	75	1.5
Weetabix	338	11.5	68.4	2

Food Type	cal per 100g/ml	pro (g)	carb (g)	fat (g)
Condiments and Sauces				
Barbecue sauce	93	1	23.4	0.1
Brown sauce, sweet	98	1.2	22.2	0.1
Capers	14	1.4	1.3	0.3
Coconut cream	350	4	5.9	34.7
Coconut milk, light	73	0.7	1.6	7
Cranberry jelly	100	0	12	0
Green Thai curry paste	100	1.9	20	1.3
Harissa Paste	90	2.3	11.8	3.6
Houmous, reduced fat (Tesco)	255	9.3	10.8	18.4
Jerk paste	81	1.2	10	5
Miso soup paste	203	13.3	23.5	6.2
Peppers, pickled, sweet	34	1.8	7.1	0
Red Thai curry paste (Tesco)	115	1.5	8.9	7.3
Redcurrant jelly	240	0.3	63.8	0
Sweet chilli sauce	229	0.6	55.1	0.7
Tahini (sesame seed paste)	607	18.5	0.9	58.9
Tomato ketchup	115	1.6	28.6	0.1
Dressings				
Caesar dressing	542	2	3	58
Caesar dressing, light	109	3	12.5	6.2
French dressing	462	0.1	4.5	49.4
French dressing, fat free	38	0.1	9.9	0
Horseradish sauce	153	2.5	17.9	8.4
Light mayonnaise	288	1	8.2	28.1
Mayonnaise	691	1.1	1.7	75.6
Mirin (rice wine)	289	0.2	71.7	0.1
Nam pla (Thai fish sauce)	54	4.5	9	0.5
Salad cream	348	1.5	16.7	31
Salad cream, reduced fat	194	1	9.4	17.2

Food Type	cal per 100g/ml	pro (g)	carb (g)	fat (g)
Mustards				
Dijon mustard	165	7.8	4.8	12
English mustard	160	8.2	18.7	5.6
Wholegrain mustard	140	8.2	4.2	10.2
Soy Sauce				
Dark soy sauce	75	6.2	10.9	0.5
Light soy sauce	52	2.5	10.5	trace
Stock Cubes				
Chicken stock, made up per pack instructions	7	0.1	0.6	0.4
Fish stock cube, made up per pack instructions	7	0.2	0.4	0.5
Vegetable stock cube, made up per pack instructions	10	0.1	0.5	0.6
Vinegars				
Balsamic vinegar	104	1.2	19.8	0
Cider vinegar	18	0	0.4	0
Red wine vinegar	22	0.6	0.4	0
Rice vinegar	6	0.2	1.4	0
White wine vinegar	22	0	0.6	0
Worcestershire sauce	65	1.4	15.5	0.1
Dairy				
Butter, salted and unsalted	744	0.6	0.6	82.2
Cheddar, English	416	25.4	0.1	34.9
Cottage cheese, reduced fat	79	13.3	3.3	1.5
Cream cheese	439	3.1	Tr	47.4
Double cream	496	1.6	1.7	53.7
Feta	250	15.6	1.5	20.2
Halloumi	315	22	0.8	24.6
Light crème fraîche	162	2.7	4.4	15
Light soft cheese	156	8.3	4	11.5

Food Type	cal per 100g/ml	pro (g)	carb (g)	fat (g)
Mozzarella	257	18.6	Tr	20.3
Parmesan	415	36.2	0.9	29.7
Pecorino cheese	391	28	0	31
Roquefort	375	19.7	Tr	32.9
Skimmed milk	32	3.4	4.4	0.2
Yogurt – 0% fat Greek	57	10.3	4	0
Yogurt, plain, low fat	56	4.8	7.4	1
Desserts and Puddings				
Meringue	381	5.3	96	0+
Sugar-free raspberry jelly	61	1.2	15.1	0
Drinks (Alcoholic)				
Brandy	222	Tr	Tr	0
Dry cider	36	0+	2.6	0
Lager (bottled)	29	0.2	1.5	Tr
Port	157	0.1	12	0
Red wine	68	0.1	1.5	0
Sake	134	0.5	5	0
Sherry, dry	116	0.2	1.4	0
White wine	66	0.1	0.6	0
Drinks (Non-alcoholic)				
Elderflower cordial (Bottlegreen)	29	0	7	0
Orange juice, unsweetened	36	0.5	8.8	0.1
Tomato juice	14	0.8	3	0+
Eggs				
raw, white	36	9	Tr	Tr
raw, whole	151	12.5	Tr	11.2
Flour and Baking				
Cocoa powder	312	18.5	11.5	21.7
Cornflour	354	0.6	92	0.7
White breadmaking flour	341	11.5	75.3	1.4

Food Type	cal per 100g/ml	pro (g)	carb (g)	fat (g)
White, plain flour	341	9.4	77.7	1.3
White self-raising flour	330	8.9	75.6	1.2
Wholemeal self-raising flour	310	12.7	63.9	2.2
Yeast, dried	169	35.6	3.5	1.5
Fruit				
Apples, cooking, peeled	35	0.3	8.9	0.1
Apples, eating, raw	47	0.4	11.8	0.1
Apricots, dried	188	4.8	43.4	0.7
Bananas, peeled	95	1.2	23.2	0.3
Blackberries	25	0.9	5.1	0.2
Cherries	48	0.9	11.5	0.1
Clementines, peeled	37	0.9	8.7	0.1
Coconut, desiccated	604	5.6	6.4	62
Cranberries, dried	325	0.1	77.5	0.3
Dates	124	1.5	31.3	0.1
Figs, dried	227	3.6	52.9	1.6
Gooseberries	40	0.7	9.2	0.3
Grapes, black/white, seedless	60	0.4	15.4	0.1
Kiwi fruits	49	1.1	10.6	0.5
Lemons (whole)	19	1	3.2	0.3
Lime juice	9	0.4	1.6	0.1
Mangoes, peeled	57	0.7	14.1	0.2
Oranges, peeled	37	1.1	8.5	0.1
Peaches, flesh and skin	33	1	7.6	0.1
Pears	40	0.3	10	0.1
Pineapples, canned in juice	47	0.3	12.2	Tr
Plums	36	0.6	8.8	0.1
Raisins	272	2.1	69.3	0.4
Raspberries, fresh	25	1.4	4.6	0.3
Strawberries	27	0.8	6	0.1

Food Type	cal per 100g/ml	pro (g)	carb (g)	fat (g)
Sultanas	275	2.7	69.4	0.4
Herbs and Spices				
Basil, fresh	40	3.1	5.1	0.8
Cayenne pepper, ground	318	12	31.7	17.3
Chives, fresh	23	2.8	1.7	0.6
Cinnamon, ground	247	3.9	81	1
Coriander, fresh	20	2.4	1.8	0.6
Ginger, ground	284	7.4	60	3.3
Mint, fresh	43	3.8	5.3	0.7
Paprika powder	289	14.8	34.9	13
Parsley, fresh	34	3	27	1.3
Tarragon, fresh	49	3.4	6.3	1.1
Jams, Marmalades and Sweet Spreads				
Apricot jam	244	0.4	60.6	0
Blackcurrant jam	244	0.4	60.6	0
Honey	288	0.4	76.4	0
Lemon curd	282	0.6	62.7	4.9
Marmalade	261	0.1	69.5	0
Peanut butter, crunchy	606	24	15	50
Peanut butter, smooth	607	22.8	13.1	51.8
Raspberry jam	244	0.5	60.4	0.1
Strawberry jam	244	0.4	60.6	0
Poultry				
Chicken breast, skinned and boned	148	32	0	2.2
Chicken breast, skinned and boned, stir-fried	161	29.7	0	4.6
Chicken, light and dark meat, roasted	177	27.3	0	7.5
Duck, meat only, roasted	195	25.3	0	10.4

Food Type	cal per 100g/ml	pro (g)	carb (g)	fat (g)
Turkey mince, stewed	176	28.6	0	6.8
Turkey breast fillet, grilled	155	33	0	1.7
Fish and Seafood				
Anchovy fillets, canned in oil and drained	191	25.2	0	10
Cod, raw	80	18.3	0	0.7
Crab meat, white, canned	77	18.1	0+	0.5
Fish fingers, grilled	214	15.1	19.3	9
Haddock fillets, raw	81	19	0	0.6
Hake, raw	92	18	0	2.2
Halibut, raw	92	17.7	0	2.4
King prawns	74	16.3	0.5	0.8
Monkfish, raw	66	15.7	0	0.4
Prawns	99	22.6	0	0.9
Salmon fillet, raw	180	20.2	0	11
Scallops, frozen without shells	91	18.3	3.5	0.5
Smoked mackerel fillet	354	18.9	0	30.9
Smoked salmon	142	25.4	0	4.5
Tiger prawns	65	14	0	1
Trout, brown, raw	112	19.4	0	3.8
Tuna steak, raw	136	23.7	0	4.6
Tuna, canned in spring water and drained	105	25	0	0.5
Pork/Ham				
Bacon rashers, fat trimmed, grilled	214	25.7	0	12.3
Chipolata sausages, raw	275	13.9	3.3	22.4
Cumberland sausages, raw	296	14.4	3.4	24.7
Gammon, joint, boiled	204	23.3	0	12.3
Ham, cooked, wafer thin	84	16.5	Tr	2
Lardons (back)	215	16.5	0	16.5

Food Type	cal per 100g/ml	pro (g)	carb (g)	fat (g)
Lean minced pork	147	20.7	0	7.1
Parma ham	223	27.2	Tr	12.7
Pork loin chops, lean and fat, grilled	184	31.6	0	6.4
Pork steaks, lean and fat, grilled	198	32.4	0	7.6
Spanish chorizo	291	18	3.2	23
Lamb				
Lamb breast, lean only, roasted	252	25.6	0	16.6
Lamb leg, lean only, roasted	203	29.7	0	9.4
Lean minced lamb	153	20.2	0	8
Beef				
Beef escalope (from fillet), raw	140	21.2	0	6.1
Beef mince, stewed	209	21.8	0	13.5
Beef rump steak, lean meat only, fried	183	30.9	0	6.6
Pastrami	123	19.4	1.8	4.3
Sausages, beef, grilled	278	13.3	13.1	19.5
Nuts and Seeds				
Almonds, blanched/flaked/ground	612	21.1	6.9	55.8
Cashew nuts, plain	573	17.7	18.1	48.2
Chestnuts, whole	170	2	36.6	2.7
Peanuts, plain	564	25.8	12.5	46
Pecans	689	9.2	5.8	70.1
Pine nuts	688	14	4	68.6
Sesame seeds	598	18.2	0.9	58
Sunflower seeds	581	19.8	18.6	47.5
Walnuts, shelled	688	14.7	3.3	68.5
Oils and Fats				
Extra-virgin olive oil	899	0	0	99.8
Olive oil	899	Tr	0	99.9

Food Type	cal per 100g/ml	pro (g)	carb (g)	fat (g)
Sesame oil	898	0.2	0	99.7
Sunflower oil, spray, light	522	Tr	Tr	55.2
Vegetable oil	899	0+	0	99.9
Walnut oil	899	Tr	0	99.9
Pasta, Rice, Grains and Noodles				
Brown basmati rice	347	9.2	71.4	2.7
Cracked bulgur wheat	353	9.7	76.3	1.7
Dry pasta, standard, raw	362	12	77	0.7
Dry pasta, wholewheat, raw	324	13.4	66.2	2.5
Egg noodles, boiled	62	2.2	13	0.5
Pearl barley, raw	360	7.9	83.6	1.7
Quinoa	309	13.8	55.7	5
Wholegrain rice	344	8	73	2.2
Sugar and Sweeteners				
Maple syrup	262	0	67.2	0.2
Dark brown sugar, soft	362	0.1	101.3	0
Demerara sugar	394	0.5	104.5	0
Icing sugar	393	0+	104.9	0
Muscovado sugar	362	0.1	101.3	0
Sugar, granulated	400	0	100	0
Sugar, white	394	Tr	105	0
Sweets and chocolates				
Bourbon biscuits (Tesco)	485	5.4	66.2	21.6
Plain chocolate	510	5	63.5	28
Vegetables, raw				
Asparagus	25	2.9	2	0.6
Aubergine	15	0.9	2.2	0.4
Avocado pear	190	1.9	1.9	19.5
Beansprouts	31	2.9	4	0.5
Beetroot	36	1.7	7.6	0.1

Food Type	cal per 100g/ml	pro (g)	carb (g)	fat (g)
Broccoli	33	4.4	1.8	0.9
Butternut squash	36	1.1	8.3	0.1
Cabbage, white	27	1.4	5	0.2
Cabbage, green	26	1.7	4.1	0.4
Cabbage, Savoy	27	2.1	3.9	0.5
Carrots, old	35	0.6	7.9	0.3
Carrots, young	30	0.7	6	0.5
Cauliflower	34	3.6	3	0.9
Celery	7	0.5	0.9	0.2
Chilli, green	20	2.9	0.7	0.6
Chilli, red	26	1.8	4.2	0.3
Courgettes	18	1.8	1.8	0.4
Cucumber	10	0.7	1.5	0.1
Garlic	98	7.9	16.3	0.6
Gem lettuce leaves	12	0.6	1.5	0.4
Gherkin/cornichon	12	1	1.8	0.1
Ginger, root	49	1.7	9.5	0.7
Green beans	24	1.9	3.2	0.5
Kale	33	3.4	1.4	1.6
Leeks	22	1.6	2.9	0.5
Lettuce	14	0.8	1.7	0.5
Mangetout	32	3.6	4.2	0.2
Mushrooms, chestnut	16	1.8	Tr	0.5
Mushrooms, common	13	1.8	0.4	0.5
Mushrooms, porcini	375	25	50	0
Mushrooms, portobello	35	4	5	1
Mushrooms, shiitake, dried	296	9.6	63.9	1
Olives, black, pitted, in sunflower oil	466	0	20	40
Olives, green, pitted, in brine	103	0.9	Tr	11

Food Type	cal per 100g/ml	pro (g)	carb (g)	fat (g)
Onions	36	1.2	7.9	0.2
Pak choi	19	1.5	2.2	0.2
Parsnips	64	1.8	12.5	1.1
Peas, frozen, raw	66	5.7	9.3	0.9
Pepper, green (bell)	15	0.8	2.6	0.3
Pepper red (bell), stalks and seeds removed	32	1	6.4	0.4
Potatoes, new	70	1.7	16.1	0.3
Potatoes, old	75	2.1	17.2	0.2
Pumpkin	13	0.7	2.2	0.2
Purple sprouting broccoli	35	3.9	2.6	1.1
Red cabbage	21	1.1	3.7	0.3
Rocket leaves	25	0	2	0.6
Romaine lettuce heart	16	1	1.7	0.6
Shallots	20	1.5	3.3	0.2
Spaghetti squash	26	0.6	4.6	0.6
Spinach	25	2.8	1.6	0.8
Spring onions	23	2	3	0.5
Sugar snaps	34	3.4	5	0.2
Swede	24	0.7	5	0.3
Sweet potato	87	1.2	21.3	0.3
Sweetcorn, on the cob	54	2	9.9	1
Swiss chard, rainbow chard	19	1.8	2.9	0.2
Tomato purée	76	5	14.2	0.3
Tomatoes	19	0.7	3.1	0.4
Tomatoes, canned	16	1	3	0.1
Tomatoes, cherry	23	1.2	3.3	0.6
Tomatoes, sun-dried	495	3.3	5.4	51.3
Turnip	23	0.9	4.7	0.3
Watercress	22	3	0.4	1

REFERENCES

1. Miles B. 'Integration of metabolism',
http://www.tamu.edu/faculty/bmiles/lectures/integration.pdf

2. Brown J et al. 'Intermittent fasting: a dietary intervention for
prevention of diabetes and cardiovascular disease?', *The British
Journal of Diabetes & Vascular Disease*, March/April 2013, pp.68–72
http://dvd.sagepub.com/content/13/2/68.full.pdf+html

3. de la Monte S and Wands J. 'Alzheimer's Disease is type 3
diabetes – evidence reviewed', *Journal of Diabetes Science and
Technology*, Vol 2, Issue 5, pp.1101–1113
http://www.ncbi.nlm.nih.gov/pmc/articles/PMC2769828/

4. Bhutani S et al. 'Alternate day fasting and endurance exercise
combine to reduce body weight and favorably alter plasma lipids
in obese humans', *Obesity*, Vol 21, Issue 7, pp.1370–1379, July 2013
http://onlinelibrary.wiley.com/doi/10.1002/oby.20353/abstract

5. Harvie M et al. 'The effect of intermittent energy and carbohydrate
restriction v. daily energy restriction on weight loss and metabolic
disease risk markers in overweight women.',
The British Journal of Nutrition, Vol 16, April 2013
https://docs.google.com/file/d/0B_rz3P5AJBUZUUMyN196NXdoWTg/

INDEX

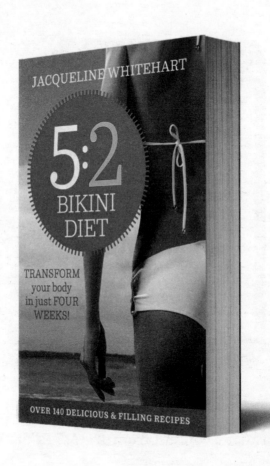

KEEP YOUR DIET ON TRACK

 THE COMPLETE 5:2 APP

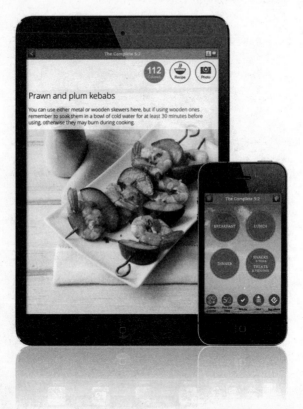

Featuring content from *The 5:2 Bikini Diet*

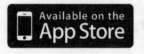

http://bit.ly/complete52diet